Diabetes-Free
KIDS

Diabetes-Free

K I D S

A Take-Charge Plan
for Preventing and Treating
Type 2 Diabetes in Children

Sheri Colberg, Ph.D.

with Mary Friesz, Ph.D., R.D.

Foreword by Jerry Mathers

AVERY
a member of Penguin Group (USA) Inc.
New York

Published by the Penguin Group
Penguin Group (USA) Inc., 375 Hudson Street, New York, New York 10014, USA ·
Penguin Group (Canada), 10 Alcorn Avenue, Toronto, Ontario M4V 3B2, Canada (a division
of Pearson Penguin Canada Inc.) · Penguin Books Ltd, 80 Strand, London WC2R 0RL,
England · Penguin Ireland, 25 St Stephen's Green, Dublin 2, Ireland (a division of Penguin
Books Ltd) · Penguin Group (Australia), 250 Camberwell Road, Camberwell, Victoria 3124,
Australia (a division of Pearson Australia Group Pty Ltd) · Penguin Books India Pvt Ltd,
11 Community Centre, Panchsheel Park, New Delhi–110 017, India · Penguin Books (NZ),
Cnr Airborne and Rosedale Roads, Albany, Auckland 1310, New Zealand (a division of Pearson
New Zealand Ltd) · Penguin Books (South Africa) (Pty) Ltd, 24 Sturdee Avenue,
Rosebank, Johannesburg 2196, South Africa

Penguin Books Ltd, Registered Offices:
80 Strand, London WC2R 0RL, England

Library of Congress Cataloging-in-Publication Data

Colberg, Sheri, date.
  Diabetes-free kids : a take-charge plan for preventing and treating type 2 diabetes
in children / by Sheri Colberg with Mary Friesz ; foreword by Jerry Mathers.
    p.   cm.
  Includes bibliographical references and index.
  ISBN 1-58333-221-9
  1. Diabetes in children—Popular works.   2. Non-insulin-dependent
diabetes—Popular works.   I. Friesz, Mary C.   II. Title.

RJ420.D5C64   2005   2004062310
618.92'462—dc22

Printed in the United States of America
10 9 8 7 6 5 4 3 2 1

Book design by Tanya Maiboroda

Neither the authors nor the publisher is engaged in rendering professional advice or services to the individual reader. The ideas, procedures, and suggestions in this book are not intended as a substitute for consulting a physician. All matters regarding health require medical supervision. Neither the authors nor the publisher shall be liable or responsible for any loss, injury, or damage allegedly arising from any information or suggestion in this book. The opinions expressed in this book represent the personal views of the authors and not of the publisher.

Most Avery books are available at special quantity discounts for bulk purchase for sales promotions, premiums, fund-raising, and educational needs. Special books or book excerpts also can be created to fit specific needs. For details, write Penguin Group (USA) Inc. Special Markets, 375 Hudson Street, New York, NY 10014.

While the author has made every effort to provide accurate telephone numbers and Internet addresses at the time of publication, neither the publisher nor the author assumes any responsibility for errors, or for changes that occur after publication. Further, the publisher does not have any control over and does not assume any responsibility for the websites or their content.

For my three wonderful sons—
may they always be diabetes-free

CONTENTS

ACKNOWLEDGMENTS

I HAVE MANY PEOPLE to thank for assisting me in the creation of this book. Without them, it would never have become a reality, and I would not have had the opportunity to potentially help so many kids avoid diabetes or its complications.

First and foremost, I would like to thank my literary agent, Linda Konner, for her diligence in finding a publisher for my book and for her belief in it, even when most editors in the publishing industry were afraid to take a chance on a book focused on the prevention and treatment of diabetes in kids.

I would also like to thank my contributing author, Dr. Mary Friesz, whose expertise in nutritional counseling far surpasses my own. She was exceptionally helpful in her review of all the nutrition-related chapters of the book, and her suggestions only served to make the book a better, more user-friendly guide.

A world of thanks are also due my own endocrinologist, Dr. M. Elizabeth Mason of the Strelitz Diabetes Institutes in Norfolk, Virginia, for her feedback on diabetic medications and supplements for youth. Her input allowed me to include the most up-to-date information available on the topic.

I would also like to acknowledge all of the hardworking individuals at Avery and Penguin Group who have helped in the creation of this book. I am particularly in debt to my editor, Dara Stewart, who was one of the few to truly recognize the timeliness of the topics discussed in this book. Without her diligence in convincing others at Avery of its merit, you would not be reading it today.

Finally, I am grateful to Jerry Mathers, who felt strongly enough about the topic of this book to take time out of his busy schedule to compose its foreword, thus adding to the book's credibility due to his well-respected position as a renowned actor and diabetes-prevention advocate. My heartfelt thanks go to all of you.

—*Sheri Colberg, Ph.D.*

FOREWORD

L eave it to Beaver has become a cherished cog of our television heritage, and I'm proud to be a lasting part of that wonderful tradition. It has been almost fifty years since the Cleavers hit town and the American viewing public was introduced to a young boy ("The Beaver"), his big brother, and their parents. That family turned out to have what every family in the United States wanted: innocence, optimism, and respectability. The pleasures were simple and the values were constant.

On that show, we were all healthy and happy, on the set and off! No one—young or old—had to deal with having a chronic health problem. Since then, my own reality has been quite different, however. I was, unfortunately, diagnosed with type 2 diabetes at the age of forty-six. At the time, I was sixty pounds overweight, and I also had high blood pressure.

By then, I had stopped doing any regular exercise. "Exercise more, and eat less" was the general advice that I heard from my physician. Of course, all that is easier to say than do when you have a busy life like I did. It was hard for me to change my lifestyle enough to lose weight and keep it off, but I kept on trying so that I could control my diabetes better.

My doctor made it very clear that if I wanted to be alive in ten years, perhaps watching my two daughters get married or holding a grand-child, then it was time to take control of my diabetes. I might not be able to defeat it, but with regular glucose testing, better eating habits, and twenty minutes of exercise a day, I could at least control its progression and lessen its potentially negative impact on my health, my life, and my longevity. Also, by modeling a healthier lifestyle for my own kids and grandkids, I might be able to help them become healthier and avoid ever developing diabetes.

Admittedly, I had lived the culinary good life since I was a child. Every television or movie set has food everywhere, and there is always plenty of time to munch on it all day long. Once I met with my doctor, I realized that I really had no viable choice but to immediately alter my eating habits from three large meals a day to five lighter ones, begin testing my blood sugar on a regular basis, and incorporate exercise into my daily life.

I've learned that being overweight also increases your risk for devel-oping an insulin resistant state, type 2 diabetes, heart disease, and high blood pressure, no matter what your age is. Personally, I have succeeded better at controlling my high blood pressure when I have been able to lose weight and keep it off, particularly when I'm exercising. Of course, everyone knows that diets seldom work long-term, and most people re-gain the weight. Little did I know that the same healthy lifestyle that I have adopted to help me control my blood sugar is also helping me lower my risk of developing cardiovascular disease, and is that ever an added bonus! Having diabetes dramatically increases your risk for hav-ing a heart attack—the leading cause of death in the United States—but even more so when your blood sugar level is not in control.

Getting type 2 diabetes as an adult was bad enough, so I can hardly fathom getting it as a teenager, or younger. This exploding epidemic among kids is horrifying to me! However, physical fitness and health experts, such as Dr. Sheri Colberg, believe that no kid ever need develop type 2 diabetes. In fact, as Dr. Colberg points out, dramatic weight loss is not necessary to "cure" or prevent type 2 diabetes in kids since even relatively minor changes in exercise and eating habits can help a lot. For instance, kids and their parents need to simply realize that TV watching, playing video games, and other sedentary pursuits contribute to obesity and that fast food joints are not the only places to get dinner!

I know from my own experience that trying to make and maintain major changes in my life to improve the action of insulin in my body (such as a complete dietary overhaul) can be overwhelming. Dr. Colberg understands this and, instead, offers easy-to-implement strategies for your kids—such as walking in place while watching TV (obviously, reruns of *Leave It to Beaver*!) and cutting out regular soft drinks from their diet—to improve your family's overall energy expenditure and nutritional habits.

As a father of three, I desperately want to prevent my own children and their children from developing diabetes; in fact, I long for the day when no more kids (or adults, for that matter) have to live their lives with type 2 diabetes and potentially suffer from its harmful long-term consequences, which often include a shorter, lower quality of life. To make Dr. Colberg's vision of diabetes-free kids a reality, together we must do several things:

- We need to help our kids learn practical and easy ways to add more physical activity into their daily routines—even if it is as simple as adding 2,000 extra steps a day.
- We have to work to improve our diets at home for the whole family, as well as focus more on our school systems and our communities to assist them in pushing for easier access to low-cost, healthier foods for our children. These changes can be accomplished—giving in to

public pressure, McDonald's even recently altered its menu to get rid of super-sized soft drinks and fries and added fruit to its Happy Meals.

• Families must make diabetes prevention and control a family affair. Mom and Dad can help by being more physically active, healthier-eating role models for their kids.

All that remains, then, is for parents, relatives, teachers, and children alike to commit themselves to making these small, but vitally important, changes to improve the overall health and fitness of all kids and to stop the obesity and type 2 diabetes epidemics in their tracks. In this invaluable book, Dr. Sheri Colberg gives us both the motive and the means for reversing the obesity and diabetes crises facing America's youth, but you have to start now—before it's too late.

—*Jerry Mathers, "The Beaver"*

INTRODUCTION

NEVER BEFORE in the history of the United States have Americans been so close to the brink of self-destruction regarding our physical health. Alarmingly, the federal government recently warned us that the combination of poor dietary habits and a sedentary lifestyle is poised to overtake smoking as the leading cause of preventable death. I would like to emphasize the word *preventable*—that means that it does not have to happen!

American youth are going to be the hardest hit by this new health epidemic. In fact, experts are warning us that the upcoming generation of kids may be the first to die *before* their parents. More than 150,000 American youth already have some form of diabetes, and at least 13,000 more kids are diagnosed each year. Although type 1 diabetes used to be the only diabetes that was prevalent among youngsters, type 2 diabetes is now reaching epidemic proportions among teens. In fact, as many as 45 percent of all newly diagnosed cases of childhood diabetes are now type 2 rather than type 1, and this staggering number is only expected to rise. This phenomenon in youth is not limited to the United States either: In Japan, the incidence of type 2 diabetes in those under eighteen has reportedly reached three to four times that of type 1.

For children born in this millennium (the year 2000 or later), their chance of developing type 2 diabetes (formerly known as adult-onset diabetes) during their lifetimes is now estimated as being one in three, and for certain ethnic minorities, the risk is one in two! Moreover, Americans are getting "adult-onset" diabetes at younger and younger ages, even in childhood. And obesity, now estimated to affect 300 million people worldwide, is being pinpointed as the culprit of this burgeoning epidemic.

In my opinion, what is even worse than this gigantic diabetes tidal wave getting set to swamp us is the fact that this now worldwide epidemic of type 2 diabetes is unnecessary. In fact, it could be almost entirely prevented! However, there are few signs that the main associated factors—the current trends of obesity and physical inactivity—are slowing down. The reality of the situation is that this epidemic is going to swamp all of us; the costs of diabetes care alone are likely to overwhelm our health-care systems in the not-so-distant future as the incidence of diabetes-related complications and their associated medical treatment costs inevitably rises as well.

This explosion of type 2 diabetes in our youth is understandably frightening. If you are reading this book, then type 2 diabetes has either already happened to your child or another that you care about, or you are at least justifiably concerned about the possibility after learning that your child has been diagnosed with prediabetes or obesity. Perhaps your own parent was recently diagnosed with type 2 diabetes, and your personal fasting blood sugars have been hovering in the "prediabetic" range (100 to 125 mg/dl), while your body weight has been steadily creeping up. Conceivably, your doctor may have already warned you that you'd better lose some weight to lower your now heightened risk of developing diabetes as well. Maybe you have also observed your child developing your physical tendencies, leaning toward being overweight or sedentary, but at an even *earlier* age than you yourself exhibited them.

Should you be worried about the possibility of you *and* your child developing type 2 diabetes? The truthful answer is an emphatic, "Yes!" Can you do something to prevent your children from getting this type of diabetes now or possibly later in life? Thankfully, the reply is also affirmative, and by reading this book, you will learn how! Take heart: If your child has already been diagnosed with this condition, it is *not* too late to prevent diabetes' potentially negative effects on your child's health simply by attaining good blood sugar control.

Preventing diabetes in most youth is simple—at least in concept. All it takes is a willingness to make small lifestyle changes to prevent or reverse the onset of insulin resistance, a prediabetic state caused by eating too many of the wrong types of foods and being physically inactive. Many people may be focusing on dieting as a means to reverse prediabetes, but that strategy is not the best one for kids and seldom solves the problem long-term for anyone.

What can you do to protect your children from this booming epidemic, then? I personally have found that the strategies that I use to manage type 1 diabetes are essentially the same ones that others can use to prevent and control type 2 diabetes—healthier eating and regular physical activity. Being an exercise physiologist, I may be biased, but I truly believe that physical activity is even more important than diet, simply because improved insulin action in your body (a beneficial side effect of exercise) reduces the negative impact of eating less healthy foods. Of course, watching what and how much you eat is also vitally important. Thus, I have used my extensive knowledge—both personal and professional—to create this book, a guide for parents, health-care providers, and other concerned adults, that can make the difference in the prevention and control of type 2 diabetes in youth.

Diabetes is truly an epidemic on the verge of eradicating the long-term health of our nation, and in order to stop its escalation, we must all learn to stop gratifying and super-sizing our immediate food-related desires. It is possible to learn, though, since doing so is not any different than learning control over other desires (such as not taking something that is not ours), which we all learn to do to some extent during childhood.

A greater understanding of the causes of obesity, prediabetes, and type 2 diabetes will help you fight back before these diseases affect your family. Thus, this book focuses on giving you the tools and knowledge you need to prevent and control type 2 diabetes in your own kids. After discussing how the obesity and diabetes epidemics have evolved, the book covers the basics of healthier eating and gives many practical tips and suggestions on how to make small dietary changes that have a large impact. The book also focuses on the importance of physical activity—in any form—to increase energy expenditure and reduce insulin resistance. Useful tips on how to add both structured and unstructured activities are given, and there is a discussion of diabetic medications and other nutritional supplements in the final chapter of the book.

So, if you could prevent your kids from developing type 2 diabetes or minimize its negative impact on their health if it has already been diagnosed, are you willing to work to achieve these attainable goals? If so, then read on . . . and prepare to be rewarded with innumerable health benefits for the whole family. Type 2 diabetes does not have to be your child's destiny!

Diabetes-Free
KIDS

THE INCREASING PREVALENCE
OF TYPE 2 DIABETES IN KIDS

TWENTY YEARS AGO, type 2 diabetes (a condition once known as "adult-onset" diabetes) in kids was virtually unheard of, and it is impossible for our genes to have been altered quickly enough to account for the unparalleled, explosive rise in new cases of diabetes. So, then why is the teenage crowd currently the most rapidly increasing group of people being diagnosed with this type of diabetes? The answer, a colleague once asserted confidently to a lecture hall full of people, is "chips and chips." (I immensely prefer his explanation to a similar one that I have heard that more directly—and likely mistakenly—accuses our children of being the root of the problem: "gluttony and sloth.") Specifically, he was referring to potato chips and computer chips. While "chips" may not fully explain this new epidemic, what they represent in large part does.

Unhealthy Lifestyles as the Root of the Problem

On the whole, the rise in type 2 diabetes in American's youth has paralleled their increased consumption of high-calorie, low-nutritional value "fast foods" (like potato chips and french fries), concomitant with the rise in the sedentary, leisure-time pursuits of our children (like computers and video games, both of which are now found in most American households). No parent will deny that a television or computer is a natural babysitter for kids when we are busy fixing a meal, cleaning the house, working late, or taking care of other adult responsibilities. Couple that convenience with the entertainment factor of the newer advances in technology that involve a screen of any sort—PlayStation, Xbox, GameCube, GameBoy, hi-tech computer games, PDA and cellular-phone games to name a few—that target our children with high-paced, entertaining action and steal their desire to be physically active during their leisure time, and you wind up with what we are currently dealing with: a society full of sedentary, overweight youngsters.

Other Contributory Diabetes Risk Factors

Not all children are equally at risk for developing type 2 diabetes, though. Thus, in order to devise strategies to prevent it from manifesting widely in specific populations, it is helpful to identify youth with the highest risk. According to the latest Centers for Disease Control (CDC) statistics, the majority of youngsters developing this condition are between ten and nineteen years of age, overweight or obese, insulin resistant, and they have a strong family history of type 2 diabetes.

The age of the child plays a role in the development of diabetes because going through puberty, notorious for raging hormones, can precipitate the onset of diabetes when combined with the unhelpful metabolic changes caused by our modern lifestyle. The hormones released during puberty in the teenage years contribute to a state of insulin resistance by decreasing the action of insulin in the body. Insulin is essential for facilitating the uptake of glucose (blood sugar) into cells such as fat and muscle; reduced insulin action may, therefore, result in elevated blood sugars if insulin levels fail to rise enough to overcome the resistant state. More girls than boys are being diagnosed. While the onset of type 2 diabetes is most common mid-puberty, it has been reported in children as young as four years of age!

Obesity—defined as having a body weight that is greater than 120 percent of the ideal (relative to height)—is generally considered another significant risk factor for diabetes development. Most obese children are already overproducing insulin. This overproduction may limit their body's ability to release more when the need arises (for instance, when a soft drink full of sugar is consumed). Having too much fat stored in their bodies can contribute to an insulin resistant state, which occurs when fat and muscle cells become less responsive to circulating insulin. This in turn requires that more insulin be released to have the same lowering effect on blood sugars. Hyperglycemia, or high blood sugar, results when this additional insulin release is no longer possible.

Family history of this condition plays a very large role in diabetes development. According to a report published by the American Diabetes Association (ADA) in 2000, 45 to 80 percent of diagnosed children have at least one parent with type 2 diabetes, and many have a family history that spans several generations; 74 to 100 percent have a first- or second-degree relative with diabetes (a parent, grandparent, sibling, or other close relative) who may or may not have been diagnosed. Furthermore, studies of identical twins have shown that when one of the twins develops type 2 diabetes, the chance that the other twin will also develop it at some point is nearly 100 percent. The latest estimates suggest that a third of the people with type 2 diabetes are still undiagnosed—blissfully unaware of having diabetes, but in the case of diabetes, ignorance is definitely not bliss! Preventable diabetic complications are more likely to develop if diabetes goes untreated.

Finally, ethnicity is a strong predictor of diabetes risk. Native American youth have the highest prevalence of type 2 diabetes by far, followed by other ethnic groups (Hispanic, African American, and Asian), and last, Caucasians. Female Hispanics have greater than a 50 percent chance of developing diabetes during their lifetimes, and the risk for Hispanic males is only slightly less. For African Americans, the risk is not much better at 49 percent and 41 percent for females and males, respectively. Caucasians have the lowest lifetime risk, with only about a third of females and a little more than a quarter of males likely to develop it. But this is still a much greater incidence than need be!

Even with a strong genetic tendency toward diabetes development, inherited traits do *not* have to dictate your child's destiny in this case. If ridding your child of prediabetes or type 2 diabetes were as easy as taking a "miracle" pill once a day, though, then there would be no need for this book. Obviously, it is not quite that effortless! Nevertheless, it is achievable with a little determination, and once you learn some basic facts about diabetes and techniques to set you on the right path, it is rather straightforward. In upcoming chapters, you will read about recent evidence that shows how a few simple dietary changes and the initiation of any regular physical activity can substantially reduce the risk for developing diabetes, even in adults with the highest risk—and even more so in at-risk youth, because of their younger age.

Role of Body Fat Distribution in Health

Adipose (fat) tissue is now recognized as an immensely more complex tissue than ever before; it is not a dormant storage depot for fat as was once thought, but rather a dynamic organ that releases its own hormones that "talk" to other parts of the body (the brain, in particular) to control food intake and energy balance. Surprisingly, though, not all fat depots are equally active. In terms of health risks, body-fat distribution (where on your body you carry your excess fat) is also important and most easily assessed with the waist-to-hip circumference ratio (WHR).

Waist measurements (in inches or centimeters) are made around the narrowest part of your waist below your rib cage and above or at your umbilicus (belly button), while hip measures are taken around the widest part of your buttocks. Jokingly nicknamed the "gut-to-butt ratio," WHR has been studied extensively because the distribution of fat deposits may be even more important than the total amount of stored fat—especially when it comes to your family's risk of developing type 2 diabetes.

People with abdominal obesity (an apple body shape, found more typically in men and nicknamed a "beer gut," regardless of its actual cause) store a greater amount of fat tissue deep within the abdominal cavity in and around the internal organs, called visceral fat. This type of fat is more metabolically active, making it easier to gain and lose, but also linking it to most of the metabolic disorders commonly associated with obesity, such as insulin resistance, type 2 diabetes, high blood pressure, high cholesterol levels, and heart disease.

On the other hand, being heavier around the hips and thighs, or pear-shaped, as many women are, is less associated with deleterious, metabolic derangements; so, metabolically speaking, it's far better to be a pear than an apple! Unfortunately, body fat patterning is largely determined by genetics, so we only really have control over the total amount of fat that we store, not where we put it. Desirable WHRs in adults differ by sex: A WHR less than or equal to 0.9 reduces metabolic risk for men, while 0.8 is the cutoff for women. For either sex, a WHR exceeding 1.0 places people in the danger zone for undesirable health consequences. The younger set's fat deposition is similar to adults, and youth appear to suffer the same metabolic derangements from an elevation in WHR.

Excess Body Fat and Diabetes Onset

Being overfat has a bad rap as far as health is concerned! Extra body fat gets blamed for everything from high blood pressure to elevated cholesterol levels and even diabetes. In fact, obesity has also been labeled as the direct cause of hyperinsulinemia (elevated insulin levels), glucose intolerance (indicative of insulin resistance), heart disease, congestive heart failure, gallstones, gout, arthritis, sleep apnea (when people stop breathing for short periods of time while asleep), some types of cancer (such as endometrial, breast, prostate, and colon), infertility and menstrual irregularities in women, and psychological disorders. Before automatically jumping on the same bandwagon, though, we need to more closely examine the causes and consequences of obesity and the role that it actually plays in our health.

Americans have undeniably become increasingly body-fat phobic. Many of us are guilty of counseling clients, patients, and friends over the years about the health wonders of weight loss, with the customarily elusive goal being the attainment of a nearly perfect body weight and shape. Nearly every medical and health organization has been on this very same bandwagon, taking the position that without significant weight loss, health benefits are not possible. Now, I'm not saying that obesity is entirely harmless and losing weight is unimportant to your family's health. I am now convinced, though, that the purported health benefits of and need for *substantial* weight loss have likely been greatly exaggerated over the years by the medical community.

The main problem is simply that for many of these health concerns (the metabolic ones in particular), the scientific research does not actually support the idea that substantial weight loss will help treat them. In fact, it now appears that many scientists themselves are guilty of incorrectly jumping to conclusions and assuming that the coexistence of obesity with these other health problems proves cause and effect, or that obesity is the direct cause, when more evidence to the contrary exists.

Generally speaking, excess body fat is more appropriately considered a *symptom* of its many possible associated health conditions, such as insulin resistance, rather than the sole or direct cause of the problem. Excess body fat is generally thought to cause insulin resistance since the vast majority of people exhibiting it are indeed overfat. In fact, over 80 percent of adults and children diagnosed with type 2 diabetes have significant amounts of excess body fat, and this form of diabetes has long been labeled an insulin resistance syndrome. However, not all people (kids included) who are carrying extra body fat are insulin resistant (more on this later in chapter 4). In fact, insulin resistance can be abated without a significant loss of body fat if certain lifestyle adjustments are made, confirming that this extra body fat is mostly just a visible symptom of the way you choose to live.

An exercise physiologist ahead of his time, Dr. Glenn Gaesser spent many years poring through all of the scientific evidence from the last decade on the topic of obesity and physical illness, culminating in a book entitled *Big Fat Lies: The Truth About Your Weight and Your Health*. In his text, he reiterates the point that individuals newly diagnosed with type 2 diabetes often can control their condition right from the start with dietary changes and increased physical activity alone, with only minor weight loss. Such findings have still led most people to incorrectly conclude that a reduction in body fat is what causes the desired improvement in diabetes control, or that obesity was the problem, weight loss the cure. However, it is fully possible to experience improvements in diabetic control *without* weight loss.

Much of the scientific evidence supporting this observation comes from studies conducted by the Pritikin Longevity Centers on people who entered their three-week long programs. Invariably, their participants followed diets that were higher in fiber and complex carbohydrates, but very low in refined sugar, cholesterol, fat, and salt. In addition, they all engaged in thirty minutes or more of daily exercise. Their results with type 2 diabetic adults have been astounding: Almost three-quarters of those who are taking oral diabetic medications (used for blood glucose control) are able to discontinue them after the three weeks, and close to 40 percent on insulin injections are also able to control their blood glucose levels without taking extra insulin. Although some weight loss occurs on such a program, their body fat afterward is far from ideal, yet at the same time, their diabetes control is vastly improved.

With regard to whether obesity by itself causes type 2 diabetes, the answer then can only be an emphatic, "No!" In, fact, based on the scientific research from the Pritikin Longevity Centers alone, you can no longer conclude that obesity necessarily or invariably causes insulin resistance, a prediabetic state. In fact, a study in *The American Journal of Clinical Nutrition* examined carbohydrate nutrition and the prevalence of insulin resistance and found that higher intakes of total dietary fiber, whole-grain foods, cereal fiber, and fruit fiber, as well as diets incorporating a lower intake of highly refined carbohydrates (like sugar and white flour), by themselves result in lower levels of insulin resistance.

Of course, that is not to say that a state of being overfat is devoid of health risks; simply put, though, weight loss—and specifically body fat loss—alone is apparently neither the panacea it was once believed to be (and still is by many), nor a strict requirement for the prevention and control of insulin resistance and type 2 diabetes in young and old alike.

Determining Obesity

Desirable weight standards are derived in a number of ways. The most common one to determine if an adult is overweight or obese is body mass index, or BMI, which is a metric system ratio of body weight in kilograms divided by the square of height in meters (kg/m^2). BMI is calculated using the same formula for children and adults, but the results are interpreted differently. For children ages two to twenty years, BMI is plotted on a growth chart specific for age and gender. BMI is easily estimated, applies to both sexes, and is more highly associated with body fat than any other indicator relative to height and weight in adults.

For adults, a BMI of 18.5 to 24.9 is considered optimal, 25 to 29.9 indicates "overweight," and a BMI of 30 or higher is "obese." Just to give you an idea, a woman who is 5 feet 7 inches tall would be in the obese cat-

Calculation of Body Mass Index

•

To convert pounds to kilograms, divide your weight in pounds by 2.2. For your height conversion, take your height to the nearest half inch and multiply by 0.0254 to get meters. To simplify matters, you can also approximate BMI by using the formula: BMI = (weight in pounds divided by height in inches squared) x 703.

egory (a BMI of 30) at a body weight of 192 pounds, while her 5-foot 11-inch counterpart would not be classified as such until her weight reaches 215. People who exceed a BMI of 40 are classified as "morbidly obese."

According to clinical guidelines issued by the National Institutes of Health (NIH), adults with a BMI of 25 or above are considered at risk for premature death and disability, and these health risks increase in severity with greater levels of obesity. Some exceptions to these classifications apply due to limitations imposed by the fact that this index is not a direct measure of body fat. Being classified as overweight by BMI measures may result from the extensive muscularity of some individuals. For example, professional athletes may be very lean and muscular with very little body fat, but weigh more than others of the same height. Lean body mass (LBM), which includes body water, muscle, bone, and internal organs, is denser and weighs more than fat; while technically overweight, such individuals are not overly fat, regardless of their BMI. (If this is the reason that your BMI is too high, more power to you!) LBM can also be either over- or underestimated in certain populations whose bone mass varies from the assumed norm; African Americans, for example, generally have denser bones than Caucasians, while Asians have less dense bones.

CDC Growth Charts: United States

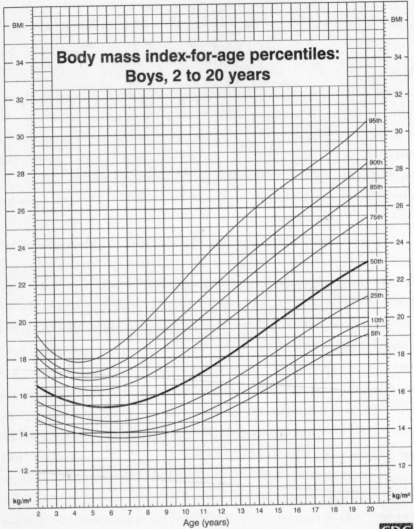

Body mass index-for-age percentiles: Boys, 2 to 20 years

Published May 30, 2000.
SOURCE: Developed by the National Center for Health Statistics in collaboration with the National Center for Chronic Disease Prevention and Health Promotion (2000).

SAFER·HEALTHIER·PEOPLE™

Personally, I prefer to use the term *overfat* rather than *overweight* since I have known many very fit, "overweight" athletes, and using the former term avoids confusion, although in this book I use the two interchangeably. For the adult population as a whole, though, BMI estimates offer a quick and easy way to estimate levels of fatness and associated health risks.

For children, growth charts are used that give percentiles for height, weight, and/or BMI. As discussed, BMI is the most commonly used approach for adults, and it is also the recommended measure to determine if children are overweight. The CDC's BMI growth charts can be used clinically beginning at two years of age when an accurate height can be obtained, and they are located at www.cdc.gov/growthcharts and on pages 10 and 12. If you prefer not to calculate BMI yourself, you can alternately access a BMI/risk calculator online at many Web sites, including two listed in appendix C.

Basically, when a child's BMI exceeds the eighty-fifth percentile for his age, he or she is considered to be "at risk" for becoming overweight. Being at the eighty-fifth percentile is interpreted that, for your child's age, only fifteen out of one hundred children of the same age and gender in a reference population would have a higher BMI-for-age. For younger children, the eighty-fifth percentile is reached at a much lower BMI compared to adults; for example, an eight-year-old boy would reach the eighty-fifth, "at risk" category at a BMI of 18, while an adult categorization as overweight (a BMI of 25) cannot be reached by the eighty-fifth percentile until the age of seventeen. However, the ninety-fifth percentile crosses a BMI of 25 at age twelve and thirteen for girls and boys, respectively, and once he or she reaches the ninety-fifth percentile or higher, your child is classified as "overweight."

Unfortunately for our youth, a specific BMI for obesity has not been established, although many youngsters are clearly excessively overfat enough to meet the adult standards of obesity. Despite the lack of adequate classifications for kids, BMI still matters in terms of their health: BMI in children is correlated not only with other measures of body fat,

CDC Growth Charts: United States

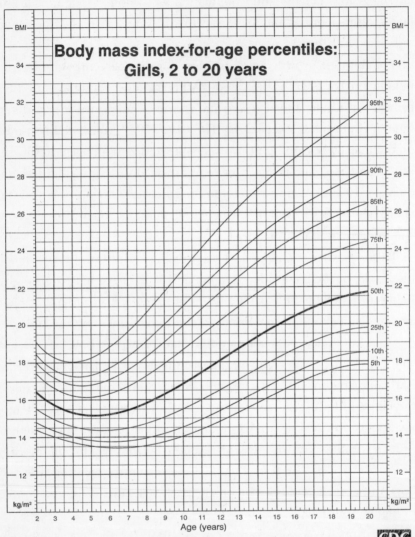

Body mass index-for-age percentiles:
Girls, 2 to 20 years

Published May 30, 2000.
SOURCE: Developed by the National Center for Health Statistics in collaboration with
the National Center for Chronic Disease Prevention and Health Promotion (2000).

CDC
SAFER · HEALTHIER · PEOPLE™

but also with blood pressure, blood lipid (fat) levels, and circulating insulin in their bloodstreams.

An adult can additionally be clinically defined as "obese" if his or her body weight is 120 percent of ideal, which can be determined from tables or charts, but again has the potential to falsely classify extremely muscular individuals as obese. For a more accurate assessment of obesity, body fat levels should be measured more directly using a variety of methods, such as skinfold measures and underwater weighing. Such measures, however, are not routinely used on kids or adults because of their cost and limited availability to the general public.

Prediabetes

For every person in the United States with type 2 diabetes, estimates predict there are more than twice as many (over 41 million people) with prediabetes. How can you tell if your kids have prediabetes? If your kids are carrying excess body fat and are inactive, they are very likely experiencing some degree of insulin resistance or reduced insulin action. Prediabetes is a condition in which glucose levels are higher than normal but not yet high enough to warrant a diagnosis of diabetes. When insulin action falls, our bodies have to release more insulin to have the same effect on the uptake of blood glucose, and if the level of insulin resistance finally exceeds our bodies' ability to secrete enough insulin, diabetes results.

But developing diabetes is not inevitable—even if your kids have prediabetes. Weight loss effectively increases insulin sensitivity in severely obese adults, primarily by reducing the amount of fat stored directly in muscle. Exercise also effectively increases insulin action in muscle, albeit by differing mechanisms; physical activity improves not only the oxidation of stored muscular fat (that is, its use as a fuel), but also the muscles' uptake of glucose. Together, these actions also cause a reduction in stored muscular fat. For older adults, improvements in insulin sensitivity with aerobic training are not always evident, but in people younger than forty years old, they definitely are—making the chances of a permanent reversal of insulin resistance from regular exercise much higher for your kids.

Though prediabetes does not cause symptoms, there are two clinical methods for diagnosing the condition. Generally, prediabetes and diabetes can be diagnosed by measuring blood sugar levels following an overnight fast. Normal fasting blood glucose levels are in the range of 70 to 100 mg/dl, and being on the lower end of the range (near 70 mg/dl) is desirable. A state of insulin resistance (prediabetes) is diagnosed when fasting glucose levels are 101 to 125 mg/dl (called impaired fasting glucose, or IFG), and diabetes is diagnosed at 126 mg/dl or higher. Alternately, an oral glucose tolerance test (OGTT) that involves measuring blood sugar levels several hours following the consumption of 75 grams of glucose can also be used to diagnose the body's inability to respond effectively to a large influx of sugar, a condition known as impaired glucose tolerance (IGT)—another marker of prediabetes.

In 2000, about 40 percent of adults ages forty to seventy-four screened using these two tests had been diagnosed with prediabetes. Obviously, the problem is serious, and vast numbers of people have the capacity to develop diabetes if the current conducive environmental conditions remain unchanged.

Since not everyone with prediabetes progresses to diabetes, you may be wondering why you should worry about your kids having it. The explanation is simple really: Having prediabetes by itself puts them at risk for other health complications, including high blood pressure, heart disease, and stroke. Time to get worried!

To more fully examine the balance between the influence of genetics and environmental factors on the gain of fat weight and the development of insulin resistance, certain subpopulations of people—in particular the Pima Indians of Arizona—have been heavily studied by researchers due to the Pimas' extremely high incidence of obesity, insulin resistance, and type 2 diabetes. In fact, researchers had previously concluded that these Native Americans were genetically doomed— over half of all Pima adults thirty-five years and older develop type 2 diabetes—and that their genetic proclivities made it almost impossible for them to avoid developing it.

However, despite the Pimas' undeniably strong genetic tendencies, inaccurate conclusions about their destiny have apparently been made over the years. Another group of thin Pimas was recently discovered in Mexico, from which the Arizona group is believed to have descended. Despite sharing the same gene pool, these two groups are remarkably different in their levels of body fatness. What is the source of the difference? One group consists of physically active farmers eating a traditional diet replete with natural foods like wheat, squash, beans, cactus buds, squawfish, and jackrabbit, while the other has become "Americanized," eating highly refined, nutrient-poor foods and adopting a sedentary lifestyle. Care to guess which group is heavier *and* diabetic? Chock another one up for the good ol' American lifestyle!

A multitude of evidence, however, now indicates that prediabetes is not just preventable, but also reversible. Weight loss and increased physical activity among people with prediabetes can prevent or delay diabetes and may lower blood glucose levels to normal; thus, obesity is *not* our destiny, nor is prediabetes or diabetes. Despite any "bad" genes that you or your kids may have inherited, it is really lifestyle issues that play the bigger role in determining whether your child, who may also be genetically susceptible thanks to you, will ultimately develop diabetes.

Diagnosis of Diabetes

So, how do you know which type of diabetes your child actually has, and can you be absolutely certain that the diagnosis is correct? You would think that since two main types of diabetes mellitus—type 1 and type 2— predominate, the two are easily distinguishable. However, this is no longer believed to be the case.

Which Children Should Be Screened for Type 2 Diabetes?

If age or weight match *one* of these criteria:

- Older than ten years of age
- At the onset of puberty, if it occurs at a younger age
- Body mass index > 85 percent for age and sex, or over 120 percent of ideal weight for height

Plus any *two* of the following risk factors are present:

- Family history of type 2 diabetes in a first- or second-degree relative
- Ethnic background of African American, Hispanic, Native American, Asian, or Pacific Islander
- Signs of insulin resistance (presence of conditions, such as acanthosis nigricans [dark, shiny patches on skin], polycystic ovary syndrome [PCOS], high blood pressure, and blood fat disorders)

When should you screen?

- Every two years, starting at age ten or onset of puberty, if it occurs at a younger age

How should you screen?

- Fasting blood sugar

Adapted from a consensus statement by the American Diabetes Association (2000).

Classically, type 1 diabetes has always been considered the *only* type of diabetes in children, except in rare instances. Now that more kids are developing type 2, or the classically adult type, it is not always possible to correctly determine the type when the diabetes is discovered, particularly because some of the initial symptoms and clinical findings are similar between the types (see sidebar, page 18). Additional markers that may assist in diagnosis are present in your child's blood; these markers include beta cell and/or insulin autoantibodies that signal an autoimmune process (found in type 1 only), as well as normal or elevated fasting insulin or C-peptide levels that show significant insulin production (only in type 2) and now levels of leptin and adiponectin (body fat hormones).

Despite the fact that clinical symptoms can overlap, how the two types of diabetes develop is significantly different. Type 1 diabetes was formerly known as "juvenile-onset" and later "insulin-dependent" because most people diagnosed with it were kids in their teenage years, although it can occur later in life, and all of them required insulin injections to survive. This type is caused by an autoimmune process set off only in people with a genetic predisposition by an environmental trigger (e.g., a virus), resulting in the body's own immune cell (T cells) destruction of all the insulin-producing beta cells in the pancreas. Symptoms first appear when only about 10 percent of beta cell function remains, but this attack ultimately leaves the individual totally dependent on injected insulin for the rest of his or her life. Without exogenous insulin, the child would invariably die.

According to the latest statistics, type 2 diabetes accounts for 8 to 45 percent of all cases in young people (eighteen years old and younger) currently being diagnosed. Many experts agree, though, that these numbers are likely an underestimation and that its undetected incidence among youth is probably rising dramatically. While many may consider type 2 diabetes a less severe condition, it is unquestionably more complex in its origin. For it to develop, an underlying genetic susceptibility must be present that, when exposed to a variety of social, behavioral, and/or environmental factors, unleashes a latent tendency for diabetes. While this genetic background is undeniably important (for example, the concordance of type 2 among identical twins of 100 percent), the unprecedented increase in cases of children with type 2 diabetes underscores the crucial role of the environment and behavior as well—most likely a combination of factors that increases insulin resistance, such as a sedentary lifestyle and a poor diet.

Many people—adults and kids alike—are currently experiencing a prediabetic state driven by environmental factors, which is forcing their bodies to produce exorbitant amounts of insulin day after day. In order for prediabetes to progress, though, the pancreatic inability to secrete more insulin must surpass the body's ability to use the hormone effectively. In other words, anyone who develops type 2 diabetes is experiencing impaired insulin action combined with insulin secretion that is maximal but insufficient. Most adults with type 2 diabetes are suffering from some degree of beta cell (where insulin is made in the pancreas) "burnout," which has led to a lesser release of insulin over time. For kids, development of this type of diabetes appears to result from the same combination.

Diagnosis of Type 1 or Type 2 Diabetes

•

Symptoms of Type 1 Diabetes
- Usually not obese (but can be)
- Often recent (sometimes dramatic) weight loss
- Short duration of symptoms (such as excessive thirst and frequent urination)
- Presence of ketones (in blood or urine) at diagnosis, with about 35 percent presenting with diabetic ketoacidosis (DKA) resulting from excessive ketones
- Often experience a honeymoon period after initiation of insulin during which insulin needs diminish significantly (or disappear altogether) for a while
- Ultimate complete destruction of the insulin-producing cells, leading to utter dependence on insulin injections
- Ongoing risk of developing diabetic ketoacidosis
- Limited or no family history of type 1 diabetes (in < 5 percent of first- or second-degree relatives of diagnosed child)

(continued from page 18)

Symptoms of Type 2 Diabetes

- Overweight at diagnosis (obesity is the hallmark of type 2, but not conclusive)
- Little or no recent weight loss
- Usually have sugar in the urine, but no ketones, though as many as 30 percent will have some ketones in the urine at diagnosis
- 5 percent chance of having ketoacidosis at diagnosis
- Little or no thirst and no increased urination
- Strong family history of type 2 diabetes that may span many generations
- 45 to 80 percent with at least one parent with diabetes
- 74 to 100 percent have a first- or second-degree relative with diabetes
- Typically of African American, Hispanic, Asian, or Native American descent
- About 90 percent of children with type 2 have dark shiny patches on the skin (acanthosis nigricans), most often found between the fingers or toes, on the back of the neck ("dirty neck"), and in axillary (underarm) creases
- Presence of polycystic ovary syndrome (PCOS) in females

Since puberty results in vast elevations in hormones that exacerbate insulin resistance, it is quite understandable that type 2 diabetes in youth most often occurs mid-puberty. Puberty is also the most frequent period for onset of type 1 diabetes as well, as increases in such hormones can overtax the ability of any remaining, undestroyed beta cells to produce enough insulin. This similar age at onset can, therefore, confound an immediate diagnosis of type 2 versus type 1.

Similarly, excess body fat used to be an almost guaranteed indicator of type 2 diabetes, but no longer. Although many of the same behaviors that lead to excessive fat weight gain—in particular, the consumption of highly refined, high-calorie, low-nutrient foods—can also contribute to an overproduction of insulin and potentially beta cell burnout over time, the presence of too much fatty tissue alone is not indicative of an insulin resistant state; in fact, insulin action can be improved with more exercise and a better diet—without any significant weight loss. Nowadays, kids developing type 1 may also be significantly overweight, and environmental factors such as drinking sugary soft drinks may simply have hastened the onset of their condition. Removing such drinks from their diet may relieve the additional stress on their few surviving beta cells and improve their blood sugars, even before the introduction of insulin injections, making their condition appear more like type 2. As it currently stands, then, the presence of excessive body fat in children does not, by itself, lead to an immediate diagnosis of type 2 diabetes like it used to.

Control of Blood Sugars

Why all the concern about having diabetes? You try to get your kids to eat a little better, avoid too much sugar, exercise a little more, maybe take a pill or two—no problem, right? Wrong! You need to worry because any type of diabetes has the potential to rob your kids, on average, of more than twelve years of their lives, not to mention dramatically reduce their quality of life by more than twenty years—that is, when they are diagnosed at the age of forty or older. If they are instead diagnosed in childhood as more and more of our youth are, then the potential loss of healthy living and total years off their lives is even more devastating!

Luckily, it is still not too late for action. We can do something to prevent this catastrophe from occurring: Controlling blood sugars in youth after their diagnosis of diabetes is the key to prevention of short- and long-term diabetic complications, many of which are physically debilitating and potentially life-shortening.

Maintaining blood sugars in a normal range requires a delicate balance among the amount of available insulin, its action at the cellular level, and food intake. Once someone has been diagnosed with diabetes, it is technically never gone, even if perfect control of blood glucose is achieved. Depending on what is assisting your child with its control, though, attaining optimal control may actually be an indicator that diabetes has disappeared, that it has essentially been "reversed"—but only as long as the assisting behaviors are continued.

For example, a recent study showed that teens, with and without diabetes, who participate in a six-month program of dietary restriction and moderate-intensity exercise lose an average of 7.1 percent of their body weight, 7.4 percent of body mass index, and 3.3 percent on their waist-to-hip ratios. More important, though, they experience a 57 percent improvement in their insulin sensitivity! The study concluded, yet again, that a huge loss of body weight is *not* necessary to see a vast improvement in insulin action. It also suggests that if you start early with regular exercise (that is, before irreversible beta cell failure has occurred), insulin resistance and diabetes are essentially reversible in youth.

Thus, a physically active lifestyle is undeniably more important to achieve than significant weight loss with regard to prevention and control of diabetes in our youth. If these youth were to continue with or increase their level of activity while making positive changes in the healthiness of their diets, they would likely experience the complete disappearance of all diabetic symptoms, and in all likelihood, they would never have to face any of its potentially debilitating health consequences.

Health Consequences of Poor Blood Sugar Control

The problem with current diabetes care is that most people never achieve or maintain optimal control over their blood sugars (with "optimal" being defined as average blood sugars in a normal or near normal range, or a *glycated hemoglobin level* less than 7 percent). In fact, according to a recent report, only 37 percent of people in the United States with diagnosed diabetes ever achieve this level of control, and so many others are still unaware of their condition and the damage it is already causing to their bodies. Diabetes-related health problems may not be inevitable, but they are a reality for many people living with diabetes, especially those who are unable, unwilling, or unaware of the need to achieve good control. With current environmental factors enticing lifestyles to further deteriorate, it is highly likely that even fewer will be well controlled in the future. Furthermore, the consequences of poor glycemic control can be physically, emotionally, and financially devastating. Poor control of blood sugar can lead to such complications as heart disease, stroke, blindness, nerve damage that might lead to limb amputation, kidney failure, and other serious health problems.

A newly released study from the World Health Organization (WHO) revealed that diabetes kills more people worldwide than was ever suspected before: currently 3.2 million deaths per year, or six deaths every minute. Younger people (ages eighteen to forty-four) with type 2 diabetes have 3.6 times the risk of dying as their nondiabetic counterparts; in fact, they are fourteen times more likely to have a heart attack, and up to thirty times more likely to have a stroke. Surprisingly, insulin resistance may be even more important to control than blood sugars when it comes to heart disease risk, as poorer blood sugar control does not appear to predict future cardiovascular events, but insulin resistance does.

Other health complications contribute more to the loss of quality of life. Diabetes is well known for its damaging effects on the microcirculation (capillaries) of the eyes, kidneys, and nerves. In fact, diabetes is the leading cause of new cases of blindness among adults, and it can cause six other diabetes-related eye diseases that can negatively affect vision, including glaucoma and cataracts. The kidneys can be similarly negatively affected; alarmingly, young adults with diabetes, particularly those with type 2, are at high risk for developing initial signs of kidney problems within the first decade after diagnosis, and some teens are already showing signs of it when their diabetes is first discovered, as high blood pressure increases their risk. Moreover, severe loss of sensation in the feet due to diabetes-induced nerve damage is associated with foot ulcers and lower-extremity amputations.

Other potential complications include periodontal (gum) diseases, which are twice as common in diabetic people. In addition, uncontrolled diabetes can cause acute, life-threatening conditions like hyperosmolar, nonketotic coma (a condition characterized by excessively high glucose levels and extreme dehydration, leading to impaired consciousness). People with diabetes may also have depressed immune function, and if they acquire a viral infection such as pneumonia or the flu, they are more likely to die from it than their nondiabetic counterparts.

Finally, diabetes in young women, if poorly controlled before conception and during pregnancy, can lead to spontaneous abortions in 15 to 20 percent of all such pregnancies and major birth defects in 5 to 10 percent of all infants born to these mothers. Poor glycemic control during the latter part of the pregnancy (the second and third trimesters) can result in excessively large babies, posing a major risk to both mother and fetus alike. So, if you have girls, their glycemic control may potentially affect the lives of your future grandkids as well.

So, you see, your family's main goal should be to prevent, reverse, or effectively control insulin resistance and blood glucose levels to prevent these complications from ever occurring. Their prevention by achieving blood sugars as near to normal as possible is entirely achievable. An added bonus is that the majority of the same strategies used to control diabetes and its complications will also reverse a prediabetic state and potentially prevent diabetes from ever affecting your kids in the first place.

GOOD NUTRITION FOR PREVENTING AND CONTROLLING TYPE 2 DIABETES

T HE CONCEPT of eating "healthy" foods was probably drummed into your mind in childhood when your parents told you that eating a cookie before dinner would spoil your appetite or that eating too much candy was not good for you, and perhaps you have carried on the tradition with your own kids. What you still may not know is that while healthier drinks and foods help prevent and control insulin resistance, obesity, and type 2 diabetes, other choices that appear healthier may actually be contributing to these disorders as well.

The food choices we make have a much greater effect on our metabolism and blood sugar responses than most of us realize. If your kids are free of prediabetes or diabetes, about one-third of the insulin released from their pancreas in a day simply covers basic metabolic needs—that is, they need this much insulin even without eating anything. About another third covers any food that they eat, while the release of the final third depends on their level of physical activity, which generally lowers the total amount of insulin needed.

Insulin release to cover food intake is dramatically affected by the types of foods your kids consume, particularly highly refined and other "white" carbohydrates, including white flour products (like bread and pasta), white potatoes, and refined sugar, as well as unhealthier types of fat. This response is heightened even more when your child has prediabetes or diabetes. So, does this mean that your diabetic child can never eat another doughnut, french fry, or chocolate chip cookie? Absolutely not! It really is not a good idea to regard any foods as completely forbidden, but certain foods should undeniably fall into a "restricted" category, while others can be eaten freely (see appendix A for a general food shopping guide).

All in all, though, knowing how to choose your family's foods wisely is as important in controlling their blood sugar levels as it is in ensuring that your growing kids are receiving all of the nutrients that they need for a healthy body. The focus of this chapter, therefore, is on understanding nutritional concepts well enough to effectively control insulin action and blood sugars in kids already diagnosed with prediabetes or type 2 diabetes.

Diabetes Exchange Diet

A good place to start in your quest for greater nutritional expertise is the tried-and-true "diabetes exchange diet," which is not really a diet, but rather more of a tool for balanced meal planning and portion control. You may already be somewhat familiar with the concept of diabetic exchanges, for no other reason than seeing food labels stating something like "2 diabetic starch exchanges, 1 fat, per serving." Many processed foods, particularly those marketed to people with diabetes, contain such information.

The "diet" includes six categories designed to group foods with similar amounts of carbohydrate, protein, and fat (known as the "macronutrients"). Often within a food category, one choice may consist of a larger serving than another food from the same list to account for their varying macronutrient density. For example, all foods listed in the starch/bread category contain about 15 grams of carbohydrate—the amount found in a typical slice of bread. While 15 grams is also found in ½ cup of cooked cereal, it takes 1½ cups of a puffed cereal to equal the same; Grape-Nuts cereal, on the other hand, is very carbohydrate-dense, so only 3 tablespoons equal one serving in that category.

Diabetes care has changed a lot over the past few decades, and official nutritional recommendations are no exception. Also called the "diabetic exchange lists" and designed jointly by the American Diabetes Association and the American Dietetic Association, the exchanges have been updated over the years to better differentiate the healthiness of foods. Most recently, the "meat" category was further broken down based on an item's fat content, as were dairy products. This has allowed users to lower their intake of calories and unhealthier types of fats by avoiding choices such as higher-fat meats and whole-milk dairy products.

As you can see from the table on page 28, which shows the macronutrient content of each of the six exchange categories, all meat and milk choices contain 7 to 8 grams of protein, but vary widely in fat content. One serving from the starch/bread or fruit categories contains about three times as much carbohydrate as most vegetable servings (5 grams). In addition, with 12 grams of carbohydrate, a "milk" serving contains almost as much carbohydrate as a slice of bread or a fruit serving.

A typical exchange diet created by a dietitian for a youth with diabetes would vary with his or her age, gender, and body weight, but it would likely include at least two to three servings from the starch/bread category (pasta, bread, rice, cereal, potatoes, corn, etc.) at each meal and another one to two at each snack (typically mid-morning, mid-afternoon, and bedtime), depending on the child's activity level. In addition, two to three servings of non-starchy vegetables (but *not* corn,

Macronutrient Content of Categories in the Diabetic Exchange Diet

	Carbohydrate (grams)	Protein (grams)	Fat (grams)	Calories
1. Starch/Bread	15	3	Trace	80
2. Meat				
Very Lean	.	7	0–1	35
Lean	.	7	3	55
Medium Fat	.	7	5	75
High Fat	.	7	8	100
3. Vegetable	5	2		25
4. Fruit	15			60
5. Milk				
Skim	12	8	0–3	90
Low-Fat	12	8	5	120
Whole	12	8	8	150
6. Fat			5	45

potatoes, green peas, etc., which are included in the starch category) would be included at lunch and dinner, along with one to two fruits. At least five to six servings from the meat category and two to three from the milk category would be included daily, while fat intake would be limited to one to two servings per meal to control calorie intake.

The primary benefit of an exchange diet is that it forces the user to eat in a more balanced manner, by including foods from all categories (except fat) on a regular basis, and, thus, its use potentially creates a more manageable glycemic response. Its main drawback is that the categories completely ignore the rapid effect that certain foods have on blood sugars (the concept of glycemic index is discussed on page 30), allowing liberal intake of refined flour and sugars as part of the starch/bread category. The concept of glycemic load (or the glycemic effect relative to the total intake of carbohydrates, covered on page 32), however, is indirectly incorporated since the number of servings of starchy foods is fairly well controlled. Everyone at least agrees that carbohydrates have the greatest overall effect on blood sugar levels and should be tightly regulated.

Personally, I grew up using an older version of the diabetic exchanges and always have them in the back of my mind when planning my own and my family's food intake. As a result, my family consistently eats very balanced meals that do not overload them on starches, meat, fat, or calories. For that reason alone, even if you choose not to follow these exchanges, it is still helpful to know the macronutrient content of a certain size portion of a given food. In appendix B, you will find more comprehensive and detailed exchange lists for each of the six categories of food, as well as lists of "free foods," portion sizes for vexing combination foods (like pizza), and foods for occasional use.

Choosing Foods for Better Glycemic Control

Nowadays, it feels like everyone wants to dictate to you what composition of foods (for example, high carbohydrate versus low carbohydrate) your family should be eating for the best nutrition and weight control. The biggest problem with deciding which foods to embrace and which to avoid is that even the so-called experts often cannot agree on what the best type of diet is. For every proponent of a meal plan that follows the latest official dietary recommendations (45 to 65 percent of calories from carbohydrate intake, with the remaining 20 to 35 percent of calories from fats and 10 to 35 percent from protein), you will find an equally fervent supporter of a lower carbohydrate one (40 percent of calories or less). At present, even the American Diabetes Association (ADA) is apparently undecided, preferring not to advocate any particular diet for weight loss and weight maintenance or formally recognize the importance of restricting certain foods, such as refined grains or added sugars, for optimal prevention or treatment of diabetes.

As the debate about low- versus high-carbohydrate eating rages on, the best approach is to realize that to choose a healthy meal plan, the overall percentages of carbohydrate, fat, and protein that your family eats is probably not nearly as important as the type and quantity of particular foods. To give you a better understanding of why this statement is true, let's take a look at the concepts of glycemic index (GI) and glycemic load (GL).

Using the Glycemic Index

The *glycemic index* (GI) of a particular food is defined as the effect a food has on blood sugar levels. As soon as you eat any carbohydrate, your body starts to break it down and absorb it; the more rapidly it does so, the sooner the breakdown product of carbohydrates (that is, glucose) gets into your bloodstream. The GI is usually ranked on a scale from 0 to 100. Thus, a higher GI means that your blood sugar spikes more rapidly after eating the food, while a lower number means that the food causes less of an immediate increase. Simply put, high-GI foods (those with a GI of 70 or more) cause rapid rises in blood sugar that are even harder to control with diabetes.

For our purposes, the GI is determined compared to the intake of straight glucose, which has a designated GI of 100. The most common foods in the high-GI category are those containing large amounts of highly refined or added sugars. Such carbohydrates are absorbed very rapidly into the system and cause the pancreas to respond with a large release of insulin, which facilitates the uptake of glucose from your blood and into your cells. A GI in the range of 55 to 70 is usually considered "medium," while a GI of less than 55 is "low." (The actual ranges of these GI categories may vary, depending on the source.)

Your glycemic response to a particular food is affected by many factors, such as its fat and protein content, the type and amount of carbohydrate it contains, the amount of fiber and nature of any starches in it, its preparation (raw versus cooked), its ripeness, and even its acidity. In addition, the exact response to a particular food can vary considerably among individuals, just like people's metabolism can vary. While it is easy to understand why the higher fiber content of whole-grain bread causes it to be digested more slowly than a French baguette made of white flour, not all GI differences may be quite as obvious. For example, the glycemic response to diced potatoes, is somewhat lower than mashed potatoes, and thick linguine has a lower GI than thinner spaghetti. Moreover, cooking of foods in general—and particularly overcooking—can raise their GI. Strangely enough, though, values for many ripe fruits (like bananas) are actually lower than their greener, unripe precursors.

Over the years, a number of myths surrounding diabetes and refined sugar intake have emerged, such as the belief that eating too much sugar actually causes diabetes or that people with diabetes should not eat any sugar at all. More recently, health-care professionals have become much more relaxed on their stand on sugar consumption. In fact, the new school of thought is that "simple" sugars (like table sugar) are not metabolized any differently than "complex" carbohydrates (starches, such as potatoes), as you can see from their respective GI rankings (on the chart on pages 34–35).

Critics of the GI like to point out that it only reflects blood glucose responses over a two-hour time span after a particular food is eaten. Combination foods with significant carbohydrate and fat contents, like pizza, however, may take longer than two hours to be fully metabolized and exert their effects on blood sugar levels. Debate over the GI of carbohydrates has led many to conclude that the evidence is not strong enough that low-GI diets alone are effective for blood sugar control or diabetes prevention.

Current research strongly suggests, however, that an excessive intake of high-GI carbohydrate foods can increase insulin resistance. Not only do such foods cause an immediate spike in blood sugars, but they also increase the release of stored fats into the bloodstream hours later due to the subsequent rise in hormones that stimulate the release of both glucose from the liver and fat from adipose cells. This extra fat contributes to a temporary, heightened state of insulin resistance. In overweight adults, such insulin resistance can be decreased by the consumption of a low-GI, whole-grain diet (rather than a refined grain, "white" diet), regardless of their degree of excess body fatness. Moreover, type 2 diabetic men following a low-GI diet (foods with a ranking of under 40) were found to have improved blood sugar control, enhanced insulin action, and lower levels of blood fats after only four weeks. In short, such positive results are one reason why I so strongly advocate using the GI as a guide to help you create a higher-fiber, more nutritious meal plan for your family.

Limit Glycemic Load

Of similar importance in the control of insulin resistance is the related concept of *glycemic load* (GL), a relatively new way to assess the impact total carbohydrate intake has on blood glucose. The GL takes into account both the GI and the quantity of carbohydrates in a particular food. A GL of 20 or more is designated as "high," 11 to 19 "medium," and 10 or less "low." Foods that have a low GL almost always have a lower GI, but a few exceptions do exist; for example, watermelon has a high GI (72), but the carbohydrate content of this fruit is minimal per serving, making its GL (4) low.

Eating a high-GL meal actually makes people hungry again faster than a low-GI/GL one. This earlier hunger is theorized to result from a drop in blood sugar levels due to the greater insulin release that typically follows a large glycemic load. Lower-GI diets also may lead to lower calorie consumption even if the GL is similar; the slower carbohydrate absorption from lower-GI sources allows your blood sugar levels to stay more constant, leaving you feeling satiated longer. For many people, a low-GI diet plan results in weight loss as well.

Type 2 diabetes in our youth can be controlled either by decreasing their bodies' need for insulin (demand) or by improving insulin action (sensitivity). Elevated blood sugar levels, however, create a greater demand for insulin, which in turn constantly overworks the beta cells. It is as yet unclear whether the loss of beta cell function over time is simply due to the exhaustion of these cells caused by their constant overproduction of insulin when insulin resistance is high, or whether their function deteriorates due to the presence of toxic levels of glucose that directly damage them. Regardless of the cause, though, for children who are sedentary, overweight, insulin resistant, and/or diagnosed with type 2 diabetes, a high-GI/GL diet would undeniably further exacerbate their insulin resistance and tax their ability to produce enough insulin.

A careful consideration of the glycemic index (GI) and glycemic load (GL) of foods is crucial in prevention of type 2 diabetes; in fact, several large-scale studies have now confirmed that eating a high-GL diet over the course of weeks, months, and years substantially increases your risk for developing diabetes. But it is even more important when attempting to achieve good control of blood sugars in your diabetic child. Fortunately, modifying your child's eating habits—away from such high glycemic loads—can help to reduce or reverse the symptoms of diabetes, as well as assist in weight control. Since everyone with diabetes has trouble producing enough insulin to cover the blood glucose spikes resulting from high-GI/GL meals and snacks, the best way to better manage blood sugars is to control both the type and the amount of carbohydrates consumed.

Achieve Glycemic Control with the GI/GL Table

For better glycemic control, it is a good idea to steer completely clear of all foods that are in the "high GI, high GL" category (shown in the table that follows). Many of these qualify as nutrient-lacking "white" foods that are packed with calories. To make matters worse, one "serving" of these items is considerably less than most people consume. For example,

Glycemic Index and Glycemic Load of Common Foods (per 50-Gram Serving)

	Low GI (<55) Food (Glycemic index, Glycemic load)	Medium GI (55 to 70) Food (Glycemic index, Glycemic load)	High GI (>70) Food (Glycemic index, Glycemic load)

LOW GL
(≤ 10)
	Apples (38,6)
	Beans, baked (48,7)
	Beans, kidney (28,7)
	Bread, whole grain (51,7)
	Carrots (47,3)
	Cereal, All-Bran (42,9)
	Chickpeas (28,8)
	Cookie, oatmeal (54,9)
	Fructose sweetener (20,2)
	Grapefruit (25,3)
	Grapes (46,8)
	Ice cream, low-fat (43,5)
	Ice cream, premium
	  (38,4)
	Juice, carrot (43,10)
	Juice, tomato (38,4)
	Lentils, red (26,5)
	M&M's, peanut (33,6)
	Milk, skim (32,4)
	Milk, soy (42,7)
	Milk, whole (40,3)
	Oranges (42,5)
	Peaches (42,5)
	Peaches, canned in
	  juice (38,9)
	Peanuts (14,1)
	Pears (38,4)
	Peas, green (48,3)
	Prunes (29,10)
	Strawberries (40,1)
	Tortellini, cheese (50,10)
	Yogurt, low-fat (27,7)
	Yogurt, nonfat,
	  artificially sweetened
	  (24,3)
		Apricots (57,5)
		Beets (64,5)
		Cantaloupe (65,4)
		Honey (55,10)
		Ice cream, regular (61,8)
		Peaches, canned in
		  heavy syrup (55,9)
		Pineapple (59,7)
		7-grain bread (55,8)
		Sugar, white (68,7)
			Bread, white flour (70,10)
			Bread, whole wheat (71,9)
			Popcorn (72,8)
			Watermelon (72,4)

	Low GI (<55) Food (Glycemic index, Glycemic load)	Medium GI (55 to 70) Food (Glycemic index, Glycemic load)	High GI (>70) Food (Glycemic index, Glycemic load)
MEDIUM GL (11 TO 19)	Bananas (52,12) Beans, navy (38,12) Bread, sourdough wheat (54,15) Buckwheat (54,16) Cookie bar, Twix (44,17) Corn, sweet (53,17) Fettucine (40,18) Juice, apple (40,12) Juice, grapefruit (48,11) Juice, pineapple (46,16) Ravioli, meat (39,15)	Cake, angel food (67,19) Cereal, Raisin Bran (61,12) Cereal, Special K (69,14) Croissant (67,17) Juice, orange (57,15) Muffin, bran (60,15) Oatmeal, old-fashioned (58,13) Oatmeal, quick (66,17) Pizza, cheese (60,16) Potatoes, new (57,12) Potatoes, sweet (61,17) Rice, brown, boiled (55,18) Rice, wild (57,18)	Doughnut, cake-type (76,17) Cereal, Cheerios (74,15) Cereal, Grape-Nuts (75,16) Cereal, shredded wheat (75,15) Cereal, Total (76,17) Crackers, soda (74,12) Gatorade, 12 oz (78,17) Potatoes, mashed (85,17) Pretzels (83,16) Muffin, English (77,11) Rice cakes, puffed (78,17) Wafers, vanilla (77,14)
HIGH GL (≥ 20)	Linguine (46,22) Macaroni (47,23) Spaghetti (44,21)	Candy bar, Mars (65,26) Candy bar, Snickers (68,23) Coca-Cola, 12 oz can (63,23) Cranberry juice cocktail (68,24) Couscous (65,23) Kudos, whole-grain bar, chocolate chip (62,20) Macaroni and cheese, boxed (64,32) PowerBar (56,24) Raisins (64,28) Rice, white, boiled (64,23)	Bagel, white flour (72,25) Candy, Skittles (70,32) Cereal, cornflakes (92,24) Cereal, Golden Grahams (71,18) Cereal, Krispix (87,22) Cereal, Rice Krispies (82,22) French fries (75,22) Fruit bars, strawberry (90,23) Fruit Roll-Ups (99,24) Jelly beans (78,22) Potato, baked (85,26) Pop-Tart, double chocolate (70,24)

GI is based on a comparison to glucose, which has a GI of 100. Information from "International Table of Glycemic Index and Load Values: 2002."

when pouring a typical bowl of cold cereal in the morning, your teens are more than likely giving themselves the equivalent of at least two to three full servings, based on a "serving" listed on the food label or in the GI/GL table. Not only that, most of these foods also fall significantly short of having any real nutritional value; they contain very few vitamins and minerals (unless fortified by the manufacturer) and little or no dietary fiber, as they are made from white flour and refined sugars.

Really, the only time that your diabetic child should ever eat one of these foods is to treat hypoglycemia (a low blood sugar)—and even then, only a small amount (i.e., a single serving or less) of any of these foods is needed to rapidly raise blood sugars back to normal. Keep in mind, the larger the portion, the greater your child's insulin demand will be. It's likely that your child's pancreas will not be able to supply adequate insulin to cover the cereal, higher blood sugars will result, and then (in a cyclic fashion) an even greater state of insulin resistance will follow.

Your kids will also benefit from limiting their intake of foods found in the high-GI/medium-GL or the medium-GI/high-GL categories because, as with the high-GI/GL foods, a typical portion is greater than a single serving and will result in a large carbohydrate intake and subsequent need for insulin. Realistically, does anyone eat only one small scoop (equivalent to just half a cup) of mashed potatoes? And who actually eats only a quarter of a PowerBar at a time or just a tiny (less than 1-ounce) box of raisins? You can help your children achieve better glycemic control by limiting their selection of such foods; if they are consumed, the serving size should be limited, as often as possible, to no more than one serving (50 grams, or about 2 ounces). Better yet, focus instead on eating larger amounts of more healthful lower-GI/GL foods, which include most vegetables, whole fruits, nuts, low-fat or nonfat dairy products, soy products, and legumes.

For the combined GI and GL of one serving of some common foods in the typical American diet, see the table on pages 34–35. Note that the serving size portrayed is about 2 ounces (50 grams), and the numbers in parentheses represent the following: (GI, GL).

Pay Attention to Other Factors

After you eat a particular food, the actual rate of its absorption from your gut may be affected by a number of factors, such as its acid, fat, and fiber content, as well as the other foods you eat along with it. High-acid foods, such as vinegar, can lower the GI of a food when eaten in combination. Even though a higher fat content generally lowers the immediate glycemic effect of a food (the GI for a baked potato is higher than that for potato chips), many types of fat are actually detrimental to your metabolism and can cause insulin resistance on their own. In particular, saturated fats (which are solid at room temperature), such as those found in abundance in red meat, butter, dairy fat, and tropical oils (palm and coconut), have been shown to decrease insulin action and result in higher blood sugar levels. Trans fats, which are created during manufacturing and are commonly found in margarines, crackers, baked goods, and other processed foods, have a similar negative effect on insulin action.

The fat you eat, therefore, should not be discounted simply because it has a low GI. While eating a large fat load may initially slow down your carbohydrate absorption, it may also make you more insulin resistant four to five hours later when the metabolized fat hits your system and reduces the uptake of glucose, particularly if you ate saturated or trans fats. This effect is why pizza—with its high content of refined carbohydrates and saturated dairy fat—is best eaten only in very small quantities (no more than one to two slices) and complemented with plenty of salad or other low-GI, low-fat, high-fiber foods. Healthy fats, such as those found in fish, nuts, and olive oil, do not appear to cause insulin resistance.

If your child is already insulin resistant, be forewarned that eating a high-GI food will also have an even greater effect on blood glucose levels. When insulin does not work properly, blood sugars spike even higher in response to eating a high-GI food or a large GL compared to when insulin is more effective. Moreover, the timing of eating such foods can also have an effect. For example, blood sugars rise more following lunch when people have eaten a high-GI breakfast compared to a lower-GI one—despite a greater release of insulin. Thus, the glycemic effect of a higher GI/GL intake first thing in the morning potentially has negative consequences later in the day as well.

When selecting the best foods for your family to eat, the best advice is to take the glycemic effect, total carbohydrate content, and nutrient density of your meals and snacks into account. It is best to limit intake of foods with both a high or medium GI and a high GL. Any carbohydrate-rich meal (one with an overall high GL) will require the release of more insulin, but at least if the GI is lower—as is generally the case with higher-fiber foods—the immediate rise in blood sugars will be lessened, and your child will likely feel satisfied longer. Keep in mind that despite the fact that most pasta has a lower GI, if your child eats more than half a cup of it (one serving), the large carbohydrate load will still have a pronounced glycemic effect, albeit delayed. Also, if he or she has previously eaten high-GI or -GL foods, his or her body may have a harder time handling subsequent large amounts of carbohydrates as well—that is, unless he or she exercises first.

Consume More Dietary Fiber

It should come as no surprise to hear that Americans, as a whole, do not eat enough fiber. Although you may think of fiber as something only older individuals need to take for "regularity," reading this section should modernize your thoughts. "Fiber" is a collective term used to describe the indigestible polysaccharides that we get in our diets, both naturally in foods and from "functional" sources extracted or isolated from foods or manufactured synthetically (like Metamucil). Our fiber needs are best met by eating whole foods, though. The recommended fiber intake for adults is 25 to 40 grams per day, depending on caloric intake (12.5 grams per 1,000 calories consumed). For children, the recommended amount is equal to their age plus 5 grams daily. Thus, the recommended fiber intake for a ten-year-old would be 15 grams (10 plus 5).

Fiber is categorized as insoluble or soluble, according to its solubility in water. Insoluble fiber is the kind found in foods like vegetables (carrots, celery, and the skins of corn kernels), parts of fruit (apple peels), brown rice, and whole grains (i.e., the outer membranes of wheat kernels). Also known as "roughage," this form of fiber passes through your digestive system without being fully digested, thus it primarily serves to increase fecal bulk and ensure regular elimination of fecal waste. Soluble fiber, like that found in oatmeal, legumes (beans), seeds, fruits (apples, bananas, citrus fruits), and vegetables, dissolves in water and is partially metabolized in the large intestine by "friendly" bacteria that normally reside there. This type of fiber may play a larger role in removing cholesterol from the body. As fiber pulls some water out of your body, it is best to add an extra glass or two of water to go along with the higher fiber in your family's diet.

While the movement of fiber through your digestive tract may not be desirable to discuss at the dinner table, the health benefits of eating more of it definitely are. A high-fiber diet may help reduce your chances of developing heart disease, diabetes, obesity, a stroke, and certain types of cancer (e.g., colon cancer), diverticulosis, and hemorrhoids. A recent study found that for kids, their fiber intake rather than their consumption of fat calories was more closely related to their body weight—and kids who ate more fiber were (not surprisingly) leaner. For people at high risk for developing type 2 diabetes, a diet high in fiber has also been shown to enhance insulin sensitivity and help lower the risk of developing it. Even a low-GI diet containing Mexican-style foods (pinto beans, whole-meal wheat bread, and low-GI fruits) has been shown to improve blood sugars in obese people with type 2 diabetes, mainly due to its low-GI and high-fiber content (with controlled portion sizes, of course).

Fiber slows down the rate at which food empties from your stomach, and by doing so, it generally lowers the GI of most fiber-rich foods, helping to prevent rapid rises in blood glucose. In addition, when food stays in your stomach longer, you feel full longer, which may help prevent weight gain, since high-fiber foods tend to be lower in added sugars, fat, and calories. Accordingly, the carbohydrates in your family's diet should largely consist of higher-fiber varieties—those with a lower GI and GL. If you allow your kids to eat a low-fiber, high-calorie snack like a candy bar, chances are they will still feel hungry afterward, even though they have consumed a large number of calories (more than they really need). On the other hand, a high-fiber snack like an apple along with a small handful of nuts or a chunk of low-fat cheese will not only take them longer to eat, but is also likely to keep them satisfied for much longer, despite having fewer calories.

It is not that difficult to increase your family's fiber intake, especially if you can commit to eating more whole grains, fruits, vegetables, and legumes. Many grocery stores have a list of the nutritional content of fresh produce, or you can look up such information on a variety of nutrition-related Web sites via the Tufts Nutrition Navigator (www.navigator.tufts.edu). For other foods, the total fiber content is listed on their labels, which will make it easier for you to choose foods that can help you reach your fiber goals (refined flour and sugar are not among them). Many heartier brands of bread contain 3 or more grams of fiber per slice (whole-grain breads are superior to whole-wheat varieties), and baked beans and other legumes contain as much as 13 grams per cup.

Before you go heavy on the legumes, oat bran muffins, and other high-fiber foods, a word of caution is in order. Do you remember the ditty, "Beans, beans, the musical fruit, the more you eat, the more you toot; the more you toot, the better you feel, so eat your beans at every meal"? Keep in mind that due to the effects of the fiber, it actually is true. The most common complaint from people who start a high-fiber diet is increased flatulence. (If you are not familiar with the definition of this word, please review the "Beans, beans, the musical fruit" ditty!) Even though your family may lose a few friends on your new dietary plan, it will definitely be worth it: You will undeniably gain a healthier body and likely live a longer (albeit a potentially more solitary) life by consuming enough fiber daily. Some words of wisdom: Increase your fiber intake gradually so that the tooting effects are less dramatic! If that strategy does not work, try a few drops of Beano with high-fiber meals or epzote, an herb also known as "Mexican tea," for gas relief.

Stick with Natural Foods

The nutrients in foods work best the way they are created in nature—that is, the way that they grow. In other words, nutrients work best in combination with other vital ones that nature created them to work with. Oftentimes it is not just the nutrients themselves that are vital, but also the synergy of their various activities in your body. Unfortunately, while foods are going through processing (for example, when whole wheat is processed into white flour, bleached or unbleached), a plethora of nutrients are stripped out, but only a select few are added back by the manufacturers; thus, processed foods are unavoidably less nutritious than foods in a more natural state.

For example, fruits and vegetables in particular are rich in phytochemicals, more appropriately called phytonutrients, which are naturally occurring substances that can prevent and fight diseases and improve the healthiness of your body. Some examples of these substances are capsaicin, lycopene, lutein, quercetin, saponins, and terpenes. It is not possible to buy purified phytonutrients in a supplement, so you must consume these nutrients in their natural form. Doing so may provide the additional benefit of additive and synergistic combinations of a complex mixture of these health-promoting, bioactive substances in whole foods that you would be unlikely to get from a supplement, if one were available. While eating at least five fruit and vegetable servings per day has become dogma, eating up to thirteen a day is the newly emerging goal. If your kids hate vegetables or avoid fruits for sweeter desserts, don't despair! A single serving is only ½ cup of a cooked veggie, 1 cup of melon or berries, or 1 medium fruit.

Experts are now also recommending that people eat fresh produce of varying colors on a daily basis. Americans have gotten into the bad habit of primarily eating colorless foods: white bread; white potatoes, chips, and fries; white sugar; and white lettuce (iceberg lettuce is pretty colorless). However, a recent book, *The Color Code: A Revolutionary Eating Plan for Optimal Health*, discusses research on the health benefits of phytonutrients and recommends choosing foods from a minimum of four color groups daily: red, orange-yellow, green, and blue-purple.

The phytonutrients available in each of these color groups apparently vary with the pigment. For example, red foods such as tomatoes and tomato products contain lycopene, believed to help prevent prostate cancer in men; the carotenoids in yellow-orange selections may reduce your risk of heart disease; green foods such as broccoli contain sulforaphane, which may help prevent cancer; and blueberries, in the last color group, contain nearly one hundred different phytonutrients and hold the number-one ranking as the food with the most antioxidant and disease-fighting power. In general, the darker the color of the food, the more phytonutrients it contains. Legumes illustrate this concept well: Black beans are highest in antioxidants (flavonoids), followed by the red, brown, yellow, and white varieties, in decreasing amounts.

The darker-colored seed coats are where most of these compounds are found, which makes sense when you realize what antioxidants do for plants. When they are exposed to the sun (which they are continually, since they are rooted in one spot), these compounds must protect the plant and its components from oxidative damage caused by UV rays. (In humans, sun exposure results in a tan or a burn, both of which are caused by oxidative damage to the skin.) Thus, the plants containing more antioxidants are better protected.

Antioxidants are the rage among supplements for adults because of their purported ability to slow the aging process, which is believed to be largely the result of oxidative damage in the body. These nutrients are even more important to kids with diabetes, however, since the majority of diabetic complications appear to be related to unchecked oxidative stress in various tissues and organs. If your kids eat foods containing more antioxidant power, they may be able to somewhat mitigate the negative impact of elevated blood sugars. In addition to blueberries, also stress other particularly potent fruits with high levels of anti-oxidants and disease-fighting power in your family's diet; these include strawberries, raspberries, oranges, mangos, grapefruit (particularly pink), kiwi, avocados, concord grapes, and dried plums.

For vegetables, the list not only includes tomatoes and broccoli, but also red bell peppers, sweet potatoes (the number-one vegetable for overall content of vitamins A and C, folate, iron, copper, calcium, and fiber), carrots (number two after sweet potatoes), winter squash, kale, spinach, purple cabbage, and eggplant. Dark chocolate and cocoa, red wine, green and black tea, and coffee also contain large amounts of antioxidants, but stick with moderate amounts of chocolate only for the kids to limit their calorie and caffeine intake. Don't be fooled by spinach pasta or sun-dried tomato potato chips, though: These often contain a minute drop of the so-called "vegetable" simply for color. To find out for sure, read labels and remember that all ingredients in a product must be listed in descending order by weight.

Key Nutrient Concept

Another tool to assist you in identifying nutritious foods for your family is the "key nutrient" concept. Our bodies require many diverse nutrients, including twenty amino acids (found in protein sources), thirteen vitamins, and more than fifteen minerals, as well as adequate water intake. To plan your family's diet to include all of these nutrients, stick with trying to obtain adequate amounts of the so-called eight "key nutrients"; if you do so, the rest will almost invariably follow.

The eight key nutrients are as follows: protein, vitamin A, vitamin C, thiamin (vitamin B_1), riboflavin (vitamin B_2), niacin, iron, and calcium. When found naturally in foods (rather than being added by the manufacturer), these nutrients are accompanied by the rest of the essential nutrients, and if you consume adequate amounts of these eight, you

Finding More Information on the Phytonutrient Content of Foods

•

Although it is currently difficult to find information on the content of specific phytonutrients in various foods, the USDA is gradually adding them on its Web site (www.nal.usda.gov/fnic/foodcomp). Currently, this site only contains a limited number of phytonutrients that you can access through the nutrient lists, such as lycopene, beta-cryptoxanthin, and lutein plus zeaxanthin (the last two, as well as lycopene, are classified as carotenoids). Additionally, *The Color Code* is an excellent source of information on most of the known phytonutrients and their purported health benefits.

should have sufficient intake of the others as well. Significant food sources for the key nutrients fall into general categories: meat, dairy products, dried beans, and nuts for protein and iron; dark, green leafy vegetables (spinach, dark green lettuces, kale, etc.) for vitamins A and C and calcium; fruits and vegetables for vitamins A and C; and whole-grain breads, pasta, and cereals for the B vitamins (thiamin, riboflavin, and niacin).

Calorie and Nutrient Density

Another way to separate out the good foods from the not-so-good ones is to learn about the concepts of calorie density and nutrient density. First, *calorie dense* foods are those that contain a large number of calories for a given weight (e.g., an ounce). A serving of potato chips is loaded with fat calories and is, therefore, much more calorie dense than a serving of baby carrots. In one ounce, you are getting 150 calories from the chips (usually over half of them—90 calories or more—from fat), but only 11 calories from the carrots (1 calorie from fat), which will also take longer to eat and take up more space in your stomach. (Remember the advertising ploy by one potato chip manufacturer claiming that you can't eat just one? Few people can eat just one ounce of chips!) The main reason fat calories add up so much faster is that each gram of fat contains more than 9 calories, while carbohydrates and protein contain only 4 calories per gram. It should be obvious, at least to us parents, that it is much better to eat the carrots if you're trying to avoid eating too many calories.

An equally vital concept to learn is that of *nutrient density*. Nutrient density relates to the quantity of essential nutrients—such as vitamins, minerals, and protein—found in specific foods. Nutrient dense foods are considered healthier foods because they contain a significant amount of a specific nutrient or nutrients per serving, for a given amount of calories. Food labels are now required to list some of the major nutrients, such as vitamin C, calcium, iron, and protein, but fail to list the other, equally important nutrients.

However, you can easily check the nutrient content of any food that you eat by logging on to the USDA's Web site at www.nal.usda. gov/fnic/foodcomp and clicking on "Search the Nutrient Database." Their list of foods encompasses more than 6,000 items, and each is analyzed for nearly 120 separate nutrients. By clicking on the "nutrient lists" option on that Web page, you can also search for single nutrients within foods. This feature makes it easier to identify foods high in desirable nutrients like calcium, iron, and fiber, along with less desired ones, such as calories and saturated fat.

A key way to pick healthier foods, then, is to select ones that are higher in nutrient content for a given number of calories. In fact, the calorie density of foods—more so than the amount of food we eat or even the overall fat content—contributes to weight gain. One maxim of a high-fiber, unrefined diet is that you can "eat more" but "weigh less."

To lose weight, you do not necessarily need to cut back on the quantity of food, rather just simply eat "bigger" foods—that is, those that are bulked up by fiber and water. For example, broth-based soups are generally lower in calories because of their high water (and usually vegetable) content. Even whipped foods may fill you up better because of their additional air content. Other "big" foods include most vegetables, whole fruits, air-popped popcorn, and lettuce-based salads (with controlled amounts of salad dressing, of course).

Hunger is best satisfied by eating the volume of food that your stomach is used to, regardless of the calorie content. Eating a smaller volume results in earlier hunger, which is an important reason why many diets fail. When people start their meal with a salad the size of three cups of lettuce and vegetables and use a lower-calorie salad dressing, they eat, on average, 12 percent fewer calories for any given meal. What does eating salad first mean in terms of total calories? A typical spaghetti and meatball dinner (consisting of 1½ cups of spaghetti, a 3-ounce meatball, and ½ cup sauce—about 650 calories' worth) would typically be reduced by 80 or so calories for the same volume of food, since a portion of the pasta would be replaced by the salad. Such a reduction may not seem like much, but in the long run you would save almost 550 calories in a week, 2,200 in a month, and 28,000 in a year just by adding a salad to your dinner, eating less pasta, but eating the same volume of food! If weight loss is your family's primary goal, just adding a salad to each dinner would by itself allow everyone to lose over eight pounds in a year!

Other Nutritional Concerns with Diabetes

In addition to carbohydrates, you will also need to be aware of the glycemic effects of other foods, which can affect blood sugars in a variety of ways. Most meals are so-called "mixed" meals that contain a combination of carbohydrate, fat, and protein, which can affect the absorption of food and its glycemic impact.

Watch Out for the Glycemic Effect of Pizza

Take pizza, for example. Of all the people I have ever met with any type of diabetes, not one of them can easily control his or her blood sugars after eating a couple of slices of pizza! While cheese pizza appears in the "medium GI, medium GL" category—making you think that it may be a reasonable food to eat—it contains a huge amount of fat, a substantial quantity of carbohydrates that come almost entirely from white flour, and bountiful calories in just one slice. Besides, few people eat just one slice at a meal, so the GL ends up being quite substantial.

In reality, the effect of pizza on blood sugars lasts a long, long time. It can cause your kids' bodies to require extra insulin for about eight hours after they eat it to keep blood sugars normalized—and that is just for plain cheese pizza! Extra cheese, pepperoni, sausage, and other high-fat toppings or stuffed crusts only heighten the effect. I always refer to pizza as one of the "get you now, get you later" foods. It invariably raises your blood sugar right after you eat it when the carbohydrate is absorbed (within one to two hours), and then it causes your blood sugars to remain elevated or rise again for hours afterward while the large saturated fat load is absorbed (which takes a full six to eight hours) and raises your level of insulin resistance. The more slices you eat, the greater the lasting glycemic effect will be as well.

As you are now aware, it takes insulin to process the blood sugar elevations that occur when you eat carbohydrates; however, you may not know that many amino acids that come from protein (fully metabolized in four to five hours) also increase insulin needs, and saturated fats (like those in pizza) can create a state of insulin resistance when they are absorbed many hours following your meal. So, a better strategy would be to complement your meal with a salad or steamed vegetables and limit yourself to eating no more than one or two slices of pizza (thin crust is better) at a sitting; your meal will not only be more healthful, but blood sugar control will be much easier than if you fill up on pizza alone.

Factor in the Later Glycemic Effect of Fats

While some people might try to convince you that fat intake does not substantially affect blood sugars, the reality is that fat content and total calorie intake do affect glycemic control—not just carbohydrates. As demonstrated by my pizza example, fat can affect insulin action in the body for many hours after a high-fat meal or snack, and it is common for blood sugars to rise when the fat begins to hit your system. This scenario is even more pronounced in people with insulin resistance and diabetes. In fact, a high-fat, refined sugar diet is a disastrous combination when attempting to maintain or improve sensitivity to insulin and blood sugar control.

Low-fat diets are not necessarily the glycemic answer, though. Such diets can actually cause an increased production of the "bad" (LDL) type of cholesterol in your child's bloodstream, especially when fat calories are replaced with highly refined carbohydrates. Not all fats should be categorized as "bad" or need be avoided. Recently, researchers showed that when a high-fat breakfast is eaten, if it contains mainly a "good" fat (monounsaturated fat from olive oil) rather than a "bad" one (saturated fat from cream or butter), then the consumed fat is burned by your body at a higher rate, glucose and insulin levels stay lower, and more energy is expended in digesting it. In other words, different forms of fat are not metabolized equally, and not all fat has negative effects on glycemic control.

Specifically, diets rich in monounsaturated fats, which are the primary type of fat found in olive oil, canola oil, and certain nuts, are actually heart-healthy and do not necessarily promote weight gain or insulin resistance. In fact, in one study, dieters who ate a daily handful of almonds lost more weight than others eating the same reduced number of calories. Conversely, less healthy saturated and trans fats found in dairy products, meat, partially or fully hydrogenated oils, and highly processed foods increase levels of insulin resistance—thus making diabetes control more difficult—and should be kept to a minimum in your family's diet.

Foods Best Avoided

With virtually a myriad of food products on the market these days, you may still likely feel overwhelmed trying to decide what foods are actually good for your family and which ones are not—even if you now know how to read and interpret food labels and claims. A basic understanding of what makes a food inherently angelic or devilish, or at least more healthful than another, is not as hard as you may think. Once you learn which foods are better off left in the store and why, the rest of the decision-making process becomes quite simple.

LIMIT SUGARY SOFT DRINKS

Go ahead and add soft drinks to your list of foods to limit your consumption of, at least the sugary colas and caffeinated varieties. Before you grumble and groan at this suggestion and down the rest of that Vanilla Coke in your hand, let me remind you that you're really drinking nothing more than liquid candy. Sugar-filled soft drinks have zero nutrient density, which means they provide nothing more than a significant number of calories, with no essential nutrients—no vitamins, no minerals, no protein, and no fiber. In other words, they are nothing but a load of sugar made more appealing with a bit of color and carbonation! Moreover, many health professionals are beginning to think that soft drinks and other sugary drinks and snacks epitomize one of the main causes of obesity and type 2 diabetes in children and adults: empty calories. These worthless, high-calorie drinks contribute to insulin resistance, leading to the creation of a prediabetic state in millions of people, young and old alike.

Virtually all of us would draw the line at letting our children eat sugar straight, but when your child drinks a regular, sugar-sweetened soft drink, he or she is essentially doing just that. A 12-fluid-ounce can of a seemingly innocent soft drink like Sprite or Sierra Mist (non-caffeinated soft drinks) contains 40 grams of high fructose corn syrup and/or table sugar; each teaspoonful of white sugar contains 4 grams of simple carbohydrates, which translates to ten—yes, ten!—teaspoons of sugar in an ordinary 12-ounce can. Other choices like Orange Slice actually contain 50 grams of sugar, or more than twelve teaspoons' worth! To make things worse, many teenagers drink not just a 12-ounce can, but rather 20-ounce or other oversized drinks that you can buy every-where nowadays. The extra 8 ounces of sugary soda adds an extra six to eight teaspoons of sugar.

Have you ever heard the adage, "An apple a day keeps the doctor away"? Well, it may be time for an updated saying, such as, "A soda a day keeps the vitamins and minerals away." Better yet, the new one should probably be, "A soda a day brings the doctor right away." The results of a recent national food survey found that people who are regular con-sumers of sugared drinks increased their chances of being deficient in every vitamin and mineral for which a recommended daily allowance (RDA) is given, including calcium, iron, vitamins C, E, A, and D, and all of the B vitamins. In other words, drinking soda instead of more nutrient-rich beverages, such as skim or soy milk, will likely increase your kids' risk of malnutrition—including insufficient calcium intake, which can result in thinner, more fracture-prone bones. Their peak bone mass will be reached in their mid-twenties and decline from there, so adequate calcium intake and bone formation is essential during childhood and adolescence.

Expanding serving sizes alone does not explain the soft drink phe-nomenon sweeping our nation, though. Due to the enormity of the mar-ket for such products, the major drink producers are among the most aggressive marketing forces in the world. Another obvious reason for in-creased consumption, therefore, is the ubiquitous and relentless advertis-ing of soft drinks and other sugary snacks that our children have been exposed to since birth. The manufacturers are not about making products that are good for us. Rather they are all about making a bigger profit! Such manufacturers target younger consumers by using sports figures or teen idols to market such products and spend multimillions on marketing annually (remember the Cola Wars?). Furthermore, they have the marketing budgets to ensure that their products are always readily accessible.

Both sugar and caffeine can negatively impact our children's ability to stay focused and learn. No one serves coffee to young children at school, but if they drink a 20-ounce cola or trendy, nonherbal iced tea, their caffeine intake will still be quite high. Caffeine is the most widely used psychoactive substance (stimulant) in the world. Although it occurs naturally in coffee, nonherbal teas, and cocoa, its presence in soft drinks is not a natural phenomenon. Its addictive qualities, however, may explain why the vast majority of the most popular soft drinks contain significant amounts of it. Say the average teen consuming three cans a day is drinking caffeinated sodas, then he or she is getting more caffeine than is found in a 6-ounce cup of brewed coffee (over 100 mg)— or even twice as much if drinking Mountain Dew, Jolt, or other super-caffeinated varieties. Caffeine can increase feelings of nervousness, anxiety, irritability, sleeplessness, and heart palpitations, as well as cause your kids to suffer from withdrawal symptoms if they fail to consume the amount of caffeine they are used to.

Moreover, caffeine has been shown to increase the excretion of calcium in the urine by as much as 20 mg per 12-ounce can, or 2 percent of the daily intake for teens. To add insult to injury, colas (like Coca-Cola, Pepsi, and Dr Pepper) contain a large amount of phosphate (in the form of phosphoric acid), which hinders the absorption of dietary calcium and causes the release of stored calcium from bones. Choosing noncaffeinated, diet colas is not the answer either, as they contain equally high levels of phosphoric acid. The triple whammy of caffeine, high phosphate intake, and reduced intake of milk should put genuine fear in the hearts of all parents desirous of good bone health for their kids.

Just as alarmingly, a recent study showed that moderate caffeine ingestion can also decrease insulin sensitivity by an average of 15 percent in healthy people, possibly as a result of the increased release of adrenaline it causes, as well as elevate circulating levels of fat in the bloodstream, particularly when taken with a meal. Coffee consumption, on the other hand, has been associated with a lower risk of type 2 diabetes in adults, but no one understands why yet, and this finding has not been directly tested in a controlled research study. Regardless, the effect that caffeine in many soft drinks likely has on your kids' bodies, though, is to even further exacerbate the state of insulin resistance caused by their huge intake of refined sugars, and with diabetes prevention and control in mind, caffeine intake by your kids is best avoided.

If your child has diabetes and needs to avoid sugary drinks, how do you go about choosing suitable alternate beverages? Let's start by comparing some drinks to see what might be the best choice. Contrasting 8-ounce glasses of orange juice, whole milk, skim milk, or sugary soft drinks with regard to their nutritional value, you will find that the calorie contents are roughly 120 for the O.J., 150 for whole milk, 90 for the skim variety, and 100 calories for a typical soda. Only the two milk choices contain significant amounts of protein (an essential nutrient), containing 8 grams each versus less than 2 grams for juice and none for soda; thus, milk is nutrient dense in protein, not to mention calcium and vitamins A and D (which are routinely added to milk). However, the juice contains a significant amount of vitamin C (160 percent of the daily value), as well as calcium if fortified with this mineral (many orange juices nowadays contain more calcium than milk). Only the soft drink is completely nutrient poor and calorie dense, containing a minimum of 25 to 30 grams of processed sugar (in just 1 cup, or two-thirds of a can).

Which drink is right for your child with diabetes in the mix, though? Obviously, the soft drink is out. Milk is a nutritious choice, but always opt for skim or 1% milk (containing only a trace of fat in skim and 2.5 grams in the low-fat milk) instead of whole milk, which contains 8 more grams of fat (about 70 extra calories), most of which is saturated (the heart-unhealthy type), not to mention laden with cholesterol. Choosing lower-fat varieties cuts down on both unhealthy fat and cholesterol intake. Growing kids need the amount of calcium found in two to four servings of skim milk a day. If your kids do not drink milk at school, encourage skim milk and low-fat soy milk as beverages at home on occasion. While the juice contains some essential nutrients, drinking too much fruit juice adds significant calories and may contribute to your child's risk of significant weight gain and worsen his or her diabetes control with its higher GI than milk. So, to balance diabetes and nutritional concerns, your child's best bet is to skip the sugared drinks and fruit juices, instead alternating lower-fat milk with plain water or an occasional noncaloric, phosphate-free flavored water or diet soda.

CONSUME LESS REFINED SUGAR AND FOODS

Let's not forget that many drinks, snacks, and foods targeted at kids by food companies are as sugar-laden and nutrient poor as soft drinks. For example, SunnyD and Hi-C drinks may contain some added vitamin C, but they contain 10 percent or less real fruit juices, if that much. Other drinks, such as Capri Sun, contain mostly high-fructose corn syrup and other sweeteners, while Kool-Aid is nothing more than artificially flavored and colored sugar water. The fashionable sports drinks, such as Gatorade and POWERade, are not much better except that their total sugar content is usually slightly less per serving.

Thus, if your children are consuming sugar-laden drinks, breakfast cereals, cookies, "froot" chews, candy (e.g., Skittles, Baby Bottle Pops, etc.), and other unhealthy snacks on a regular basis, their healthful calorie sources (such as whole fruits, vegetables, and low-fat dairy products) are being replaced with ones that are almost completely devoid of nutritional value. Keep in mind that almost all foods that have been processed have lost a substantial quantity of their naturally occurring nutrients. Anything made with white sugar, white flour, white rice, or other overprocessed grains will almost invariably be nutrient poor,

The Great American Consumption of Soft Drinks

•

Americans have actually known for a long time that drinking or eating too much sugar is supposed to be bad for us. Back in 1942, when the production of soft drinks began, people drank an average of five cans per month per person. Even back then, the American Medical Association (AMA) recommended that sweetened carbonated beverages and all forms of candy be restricted due to their low nutritional value. Yet, more than sixty years later, our soft drink consumption has skyrocketed more than nine times to an average of fifty cans per person every month. Even though 24 percent of this amount consists of artificially sweetened, diet sodas (which were nonexistent in 1942), sugared soft drinks provide the biggest single source of refined sugars in the current American diet, accounting for more than one-third of all the added sugars we consume.

More distressing still, our children—our teens in particular—consume *more* than their fair share of these drinks. A recent report from the Center for Science in the Public Interest reported that the average teenage male consumes 868 12-ounce cans of sugar-filled soft drinks per year (the equivalent of almost three cans daily), more than twice as much as twenty-five years ago. The average teen girl consumes slightly fewer cans. These statistics do not even include their consumption of sugary fruit drinks, fruit cocktails, and sports drinks. Keep in mind that a drink with 10 percent fruit juice contains only 1 ounce out of 10 that is actually juice; the other 9 ounces are nothing but colored sugar water!

So, why exactly do our children drink so many sodas and other sugary drinks anyway? One undeniable reason for our increased soda consumption is the steady increase in the size of soft drink servings over the years. In the 1950s, the standard serving for Coca-Cola was the 6.5-ounce bottle, followed later by the 12-ounce aluminum can. Currently, the standard size can is in the process of being outnumbered by the 20-

ounce plastic bottle (not to mention the 64-ounce Double Gulp at 7-Eleven convenience stores). Yet, the serving size on such drinks' labels still states 8 ounces as the serving size! One fact about these ever-expanding containers is true: The larger the container, the more people are likely to drink, especially if they consider it to be a "single serving" size, and Americans today are all focused on getting the best value for their money.

calorie dense, and glucose raising. These unhealthy foods increase your family's risk for obesity and insulin resistance, and they make control of diagnosed diabetes infinitely harder. Such foods are best avoided, or at least they should be severely limited in your kids' diets.

Consumer Nutritional Tools

You already know that consuming too much sugar is not good and that your kids should eat more fruits and vegetables, but what about all the other not so clear-cut choices out there? It's a confusing world now that the majority of food labels try to stress the worth of their products. Some products are "enriched" with various nutrients (like Wonder bread), while others are "fortified with a complete day's worth of 20 essential vitamins and minerals" (like many breakfast cereals). As you walk down the grocery aisle you will likely see Quaker Oats asserting that eating oatmeal "may help lower your blood cholesterol" and Aunt Jemima's pancake mix claiming to be "a good source of calcium and iron." Some foods claim to be naturally fat free, while others claim to be good for a low-carbohydrate diet. So, how can you truly know which foods are better for your family and which are not? Read on, and hopefully the clashing worlds of commercial marketing and nutrition will become a little clearer.

Be Careful When Using the Food Guide Pyramid

Schoolchildren are routinely being taught to follow the Food Guide Pyramid (created by the U.S. Department of Agriculture, or USDA) to guide them in making appropriate daily food choices. It depicts the food groups as a pyramid, with the idea being that the larger base visually depicts the food group that the USDA thinks we should choose our foods from most often, the bread, cereal, rice, and pasta group. Already, problems with these guidelines should be apparent to the savvy reader as this food group includes not only all grain products (with no mention of their fiber content), but also highly refined, lower-nutrient items like croissants, doughnuts, and pastries.

Above the base, the pyramid continues upward with fewer daily servings of fruits and vegetables, followed by the milk, yogurt, and cheese group (dairy), the meat, poultry, fish, dry beans, eggs, and nuts group (protein sources), and ending with the group we are supposed to use sparingly—fats, oils, and sweets. This top group includes foods high in fat (hidden or otherwise) such as butter, margarine, salad dressings, mayonnaise, oils, cream, gravy, as well as high-sugar foods like candy, soft drinks, fruit drinks, jelly, syrup, gelatin, desserts, sugar, and honey.

Unfortunately, fewer than 20 percent of our youth eat the recommended minimum intake of five servings of fruits and vegetables every day, a pattern that is mirrored in the adult population; in 2000, only 19 percent of men and 27 percent of women reported eating five such servings daily. Nutritionally compromised white potatoes and iceberg lettuce make up a large proportion of our kids' already meager vegetable consumption (along with white onions and processed tomatoes). To make matters worse, more than 60 percent of young people eat more than the recommended amount of fat daily—most of it saturated, trans, or polyunsaturated—and these guidelines do not differentiate between healthier fats found in nuts and olives and these unhealthier ones.

Even if you follow the recommendations closely, this pyramid can easily lead you into eating a diet that promotes poor health, heart dis-

Serving Sizes and Recommended Number of Pyramid Servings by Age				
Food Group	Serving Size	Age 2 to 4 (Toddler)	Age 5 and 6 (Prepubescent)	Age 11 to 18 (Puberty)
Grains	1 slice bread, ½ cup cooked cereal, rice, or pasta, 1 oz ready-to-eat cereal	6–12 servings	6–12 servings	8–12 servings, at least from whole grains
Fruit/Vegetables	½ cup cooked or raw, 1 cup leafy raw, 1 medium fruit, ¾ cup juice, ¼ cup dried fruit	At least 5 colorful servings	At least 5 colorful servings	At least 5 colorful servings (preferably 8–10)
Milk/Dairy	1 cup milk, yogurt, 1.5 oz cheese, 2 oz processed cheese	3–5 servings (4 oz)	3–5 servings (8 oz)	3–5 servings (8 oz)
Meat/Legumes	2–3 oz meat, fish, poultry, 1 Tbsp PB or ⅓ cup nuts, ½ cup legumes, 1 egg	2 servings (2 oz each)	3–4 servings (2 oz each)	3–4 servings (2–4 oz each)
Fats/Oils/Sweets	None designated by pyramid	No more than 3 Tsp fats/oils	No more than 3 Tbsp fats/oils	No more than 3 Tbsp fats/oils

ease, certain types of cancer, obesity, insulin resistance, and diabetes. The GI and GL of the carbohydrates that you can pick, such as white bread, mashed potatoes, or white rice, can be equivalent to refined sugar. In diabetic meal planning, nutritionists do not regard corn and potatoes as vegetables, but rather starches that greatly affect insulin needs. (Personally, I would never consider potato chips a "vegetable," but the pyramid places chips and french fries there.)

Recently, a federal advocacy panel recommended that the pyramid become wider in the fruits and vegetables section—by increasing daily intake from the current five to nine total servings up to five to thirteen. These new recommendations (released early in 2005) also urge people to consume more fiber, so if other such revisions are implemented, there may be hope for the pyramid yet. In its current form, though, the Food Guide Pyramid is truly not the best tool to use to achieve balanced and healthy eating in a diabetic or prediabetic child.

Learn to Understand Food Labels

Using food labels, the food companies are fighting for your purchase; thus, they all try to have more "bells and whistles" than their competitors. The packages may speak loudly, but often the messages are useless, with the claims meaning absolutely nothing. If most products were really as good as they claimed, we would probably not have to be convinced to buy them. Rather, we would search high and low for them in the store on our own. The burden thus falls on us to be responsible, informed consumers.

A good deal of useful information can be gleaned from food labels, nevertheless. First, the ingredient list included on the package has to list all included ingredients in descending order by weight; hence, the first item listed is what the product contains the most of, the second one listed is the second most abundant ingredient, and so on. Be careful, though: As a result, manufacturers have become adept at "hiding" high sugar and fat contents of foods by adding in smaller amounts of a number of different types of sugar or fat, which then no longer qualify to be listed first or near the top of the ingredient list. Watch out for essentially equivalent types of added sugar: sucrose, dextrose, high-fructose corn syrup, corn syrup, glucose, fructose (the simple sugar in fruit), maltose, levulose, honey, brown sugar, and molasses. Fats can be disguised in a number of forms, including oil, palm, coconut, or palm kernel oil, mono- and diglycerides, stearate, palmitate, lard, vegetable shortening, and hydrogenated or partially hydrogenated oils. Types of liquid oils, including corn, safflower, soybean, peanut, olive, and canola, are often collectively referred to as vegetable oils.

Learning how to read food labels is also extremely important in helping you make wise food choices. Almost all processed foods in the grocery store list nutrition information on the package in a section called the "nutrition facts." Foods that are exempt from the label include those that are in very small packages, prepared in the store, or made by small manufacturers. As shown in the following sample label, the nutrition facts tell you the serving size and the amount of various nutrients, including total fat, saturated fat, total carbohydrate, fiber, "sugars," cholesterol, sodium, and protein per serving. Labels will soon be improved to include trans fat content (by 2006), and "sugars" will be changed to "added sugars" to differentiate between simple sugars that naturally occur in foods (like fructose in fruit, which is more healthy) and refined sugars that are added to products by manufacturers (which are less healthy).

There are several other points to keep in mind when reading such labels. At the top, you will see the serving size and the number of servings per container. Oftentimes, you may eat the entire contents of a package and think that you have consumed only the number of calories listed on the label, but don't be fooled: The information on the label is for a single serving, *not* necessarily for the package's total contents, so make certain you read how many servings are included. If you eat two of the servings listed on the label, you would need to double *all* the numbers in the nutrition facts. For example, if you ate 2 cups of chili with beans instead of 1 cup (1 cup being the listed serving size), you would have consumed 520 calories, not just 260, as well as a total of 44 grams of carbohydrate, 18 grams of fat, 50 grams of protein, and over 2,000 mg of sodium (and the current recommendation is to consume no more than 1,500 mg daily).

The "% daily value" now listed on food labels is intended to give the consumer an indication how much of a specific nutrient one serving of food contains compared to typical adult recommendations for the whole day. The percentage is based on a 2,000-calorie diet. If you need more or fewer calories, then your daily values (DV) would be different. This information is a useful tool to check whether a food is high or low in a certain nutrient such as fat or fiber. A product is considered a good

Chili with Beans

Nutrition Facts	
Serving size: 1 cup (253 g) Servings per container: 2	
Amount per serving	
Calories 260	Calories from fat 72
	% Daily Value
Total fat 8g	13%
Saturated fat 3g	17%
Trans fat 0g	
Cholesterol 130 mg	44%
Sodium 1010 mg	42%
Total Carbohydrate 22g	7%
Dietary fiber 9g	36%
Sugars 4g	
Protein 25g	

source of a particular nutrient if one serving provides 10 to 19 percent of the DV, high if it contains 20 percent or more of the DV, or low in that nutrient if the DV is 5 percent or less.

Learn to Interpret Manufacturers' Food Claims

What about all of the manufacturers' claims on their products? You may see the claim "less sodium" on some cans of chili and beans, but how do you know how much "less" actually is? In this example, the claim means that the product contains at least 25 percent less sodium than the regular version. Still confused by what exactly are the differences among other claims, such as "sodium-free," "very low sodium," "low-sodium," "reduced sodium" and "less sodium"? You are not alone! Interpreting these claims on your own can be problematic as they are similar, but different in meaning.

Believe it or not, these claims are actually regulated by the U.S. Food and Drug Administration (FDA), which only allows certain claims to be made when the product meets its specific guidelines. Here's what the allowed claims for various categories currently mean:

Calories	
Calorie-free	Less than 5 calories per serving
Low-calorie	40 calories or less per serving

Fat	
Fat-free	Less than 0.5 g of fat or saturated fat per serving
Saturated-fat-free	Less than 0.5 g of saturated fat and less than 0.5 g of trans-fatty acids
Low-fat	3 g or less of total fat
Low saturated fat	1 g or less of saturated fat
Reduced-fat or less fat	At least 25% less fat than the regular version

Sodium	
Sodium-free or salt-free	Less than 5 mg of sodium per serving
Very low sodium	35 mg of sodium or less
Low-sodium	140 mg of sodium or less
Reduced-sodium or less sodium	At least 25% less sodium than the regular version

Cholesterol	
Cholesterol-free	Less than 2 mg per serving
Low cholesterol	20 mg or less
Reduced-cholesterol or less cholesterol	At least 25% less cholesterol than the regular version

Sugar	
Sugar-free	Less than 0.5 grams g of sugar per serving
Reduced-sugar	At least 25% less sugar per serving than the regular version

Fiber	
High-fiber	5 g or more of fiber per serving
Good source of fiber	2.5 g to 4.9 g of fiber per serving

Did you happen to notice that an entire category of food is missing? Yes, you guessed it: carbohydrates—the one most relevant to good glycemic control in your diabetic child. The proliferation of carbohydrate claims on food labels and menus desperately needs regulation. Currently, the FDA does not have any defined guidelines with regard to claims of "low-carb," "reduced-carb," "carb-free," or any other type of "carb" for that matter. Surging ahead of the FDA's ability to regulate manufacturers' claims, the recent "low-carb" craze has left consumers confused, misinformed, and carbohydrate phobic. Since the FDA has yet to define "low-carb," "reduced-carb," or "carb-free," the agency has made these claims illegal for the time being. To get around this snag, manufacturers have instead begun to flood supermarkets with products labeled with "carb smart," "carb aware," "carb sense," as well as the completely incomprehensible "net carbs." Consumers buy such products to get fewer carbohydrates (and calories), but in reality, they may not be.

To come up with lower carbohydrate levels on their labels, companies have subtracted out fiber, sugar alcohols, and other carbohydrates that supposedly have a minimal impact on blood sugar, but does a so-called "controlled" carbohydrate that does not raise blood sugar rapidly no longer count? Absolutely not! A product having a minimal impact on your blood sugar does not necessarily mean that it also has a minimal impact on your body weight; likewise, a product that claims to have lower levels of "impact carbs" does not always contains fewer calories. Most pasta already has a slower glycemic effect, but the calories (unfortunately) still count.

The FDA desperately needs to prohibit the use of so-called "net carbs" and "impact carbs," which are completely misleading claims. The number of "net carbs" a product contains is typically derived by subtracting the carbohydrates from fiber (indigestible) and sugar alcohols (not well absorbed) from the total carbohydrate content; however, the results can be very deceptive. Just to give you one example, in our neighborhood grocery store, I recently found two varieties of pasta claiming to have lower carbohydrate contents. The Mueller's brand claims that it contains "½ the carbs" of the regular penne rigate per serving, although it still contains 31 grams of carbohydrate instead of 41 (like the regular variety), as well as 12 grams of dietary fiber. The absorbable carbohydrate content is actually 31 grams minus the 12 grams of indigestible fiber, or indeed half the content of the original product as it claims. The other brand (Dreamfields), though, claims to contain only "5 grams of digestible carbs" even though it actually contains 42 grams of carbohydrate—which is slightly more than normal pasta! Furthermore, this new product contains only 4 grams of fiber (versus 2 grams in the regular variety). It claims that the other 37 grams are "controlled carbs," or ones that are more slowly absorbed, with a lesser impact on blood sugar levels; while this claim is truthful, these 37 grams of slow-release carbohydrate are still absorbed and utilized at some point, and they amount to almost 150 calories worth of carbohydrate that certainly cannot be discounted or ignored, particularly by your diabetic child!

The Skinny on Artificial Sweeteners

•

Artificial sweeteners such as NutraSweet or Splenda help reduce or completely eliminate the calorie content from added sugars. In fact, most dietitians consider such low-calorie sweeteners to be "free foods" because they make food taste sweet, but they have almost no calories or effect on blood sugar levels. In fact, in meal planning, they do not count as a carbohydrate, fat, or any other exchange. A number of artificial sweeteners have been approved for use by the FDA and likewise endorsed by the American Diabetes Association as safe for use. All of these low-calorie sweeteners may help people who are overweight or have diabetes to reduce calories and stick to a healthy meal plan. In addition, these sweeteners are useful for reducing intake of higher-GI carbohydrates when used in place of sugar in coffee, tea, or cereal, and on fruit. They currently include saccharin, aspartame, acesulfame potassium, sucralose, neotame, and tagatose, although new substitutes are being tested and approved all of the time.

Saccharin: This artificial sweetener (found in Sweet'n Low, in the pink packets) was the first one approved for use by the FDA and the first to appear in "diet" sodas like Tab. Unable to be metabolized by our bodies, saccharin can be used in minute amounts in both hot and cold foods to make them sweeter. Large amounts of saccharin have been found to cause cancerous tumors in laboratory animals (rats), but apparently not in the case of humans, or so the National Institute of Health (NIH) asserts. However, one study conducted recently by the National Cancer Institute noted that "heavy" saccharin users may have an increased risk of bladder cancer; thus, using it over an extended period of time may be unsafe. Nevertheless, Congress has removed the requirement for warning notices on products containing this sweetener. If you have any concerns about its use, pick from one of the alternatives.

Aspartame: Aspartame (trade name Equal, in the blue packets, or NutraSweet) is a widely used, low-calorie sweetener; only a small amount is needed to sweeten food. Unfortunately, though, high temperature can degrade it when added to most foods, so check the sweetener's label for guidelines when using it in recipes. Over time, it also loses its sweetness (check the date on products containing it). Some individuals appear to be sensitive to this sweetener, which mainly causes headaches, but not brain tumors as some have asserted, and is best avoided if symptoms arise when it is consumed. Also, people with the rare disease phenylketonuria (PKU) should not consume any phenylalanine, which is a major component of aspartame (synthesized from phenylalanine and aspartic acid).

Acesulfame potassium: Also known as acesulfame-K (or Sweet One), this sweetener has been approved for human use, although many feel that its safety has been inadequately tested. It can be used in all baking and cooking, but in some cases the texture of baked goods is not the same as with sugar. To improve the texture, you might need to add some sugar. Follow the label's guidelines for the best results. If you have any concerns about its safety, you may choose to avoid products containing it until it has been better tested.

Sucralose: The newest sweetener to hit the market, sucralose (Splenda, in the yellow packets) can be used anytime in place of sugar, including in beverages, baked goods, and processed foods, although you still may need to add some table sugar to recipes to improve texture. A chemical combination of sucrose (table sugar) and chlorine, its "made from sugar" slogan is technically true, but misleading. It is low calorie because it is not metabolized. Having passed all safety tests in animals, sucralose is now commonly added to many diet drinks and other consumables instead of aspartame.

Neotame: Neotame is synthetically derived from a combination of aspartic acid and phenylalanine, the same two amino acids used to make aspartame. However, unlike aspartame, the bond between the two in this new sweetener is harder to break down, so it is more stable. Only tiny amounts are needed to sweeten foods, and it cannot be metabolized by our bodies. Phenylalanine is not released from neotame; thus, it is not toxic to people with PKU. This sweetener is so new that it has yet to appear in any foods, but human studies of its use to date have raised absolutely no safety concerns and it is not known if anyone is sensitive to it.

Tagatose: Also known as naturlose, it is a form of sugar manufactured from lactose (milk sugar). Unlike sugar, it cannot be digested by enzymes in the intestines, so the most common side effects of its use are flatulence, bloating, and nausea. Although it appears to be safe to use, tagatose is also so new that it is only currently found in one food: Diet Pepsi Slurpees sold at 7-Eleven.

Benefit from ADA-Approved Food Claims

If a food is devoid of or contains less of a certain maligned nutrient— such as sugar, sodium, carbohydrate, or fat—is it necessarily healthier? Not always. Some may be lower in calories, but more often than not, when one nutrient is removed (such as fat), it is replaced with another (such as added sugars). Such changes can create problems for people with special nutritional concerns, such as youth with insulin resistance or diabetes. The following are some extra tips for all people with diabetes to interpret claims on food labels, compliments of the American Diabetes Association (ADA):

- A "free food" is one with less than 20 calories and 5 grams of carbohydrate per serving. Examples include diet soft drinks, sugar-free gelatin dessert, sugar-free Popsicles, sugarless gum, and sugar-free syrup. (Consult the list of "free foods" in appendix B for more suggestions.)
- "Sugar-free" does not mean carbohydrate-free! Compare the total

carbohydrate content of a sugar-free food with that of the standard product. If there is a big difference in carbohydrate content between the two foods, you may want to buy the sugar-free food. If there is little difference in the total grams of carbohydrate between the two foods, choose the one you want based on price and taste. Make sure to read the label carefully to make the best choice.

- "No sugar added" foods do not have any form of sugar added during processing or packaging and do not contain high-sugar ingredients. Remember, they may still be high in carbohydrate, though, so you have to check the label.

"Fat-free" foods can be higher in carbohydrate content and contain almost the same number of calories as the foods they replace. One good example of this is fat-free cookies—guaranteed to raise the blood sugar of any diabetic child with their high content of added sugars! In short, fat-free foods are not necessarily a better choice than the standard product, so read your labels carefully.

This chapter has laid the foundation for understanding healthier eating and achieving better glycemic control. Half the battle is getting through all of the marketing hype out there and really, truly understanding nutritional basics. Hurry ahead to the next chapter, though, for some helpful hints and strategies to get your kids to eat well under a variety of circumstances.

Dieting and Youth

•

An alarming number of youngsters already worry excessively about their body weight. More than 50 percent of girls between the ages of ten and twelve (not even in high school yet!) express concerns about their weight and appearance, have already been on a diet, and/or routinely characterize food as "good" or "bad," "allowable" or "fattening," and so on. In fact, even children as young as four years old are aware of body image, and even at that age, some may feel that they are not measuring up to the ideal. These unreasonable concerns are largely the result of the media idealizing unrealistic body images in ads, TV shows, and movies that kids watch, but may also result in part from their parents' attitudes about physical beauty.

Unfortunately, overweight youth (diabetic or not) who diet to control their weight may actually gain weight in the long run, according to the latest research. In nine- to fourteen-year-old overweight boys and girls, more girls than boys are currently dieting. In both sexes, however, binge eating is more common among dieters, particularly following a period during which they had restricted their intake of calories. During the three-year follow-up, children who made prior attempts to diet actually end up gaining more weight than the nondieters. In other words, their attempts to diet are not only ineffective, but they also commonly result in additional weight gain and disordered eating patterns among these youth. Forcing a restrictive diet on a child can lead to a loss of self-confidence, self-esteem, and a poor sense of self. These emotions, combined with early obsessions with food and a distorted body image, can contribute to setting up these youth for "yo-yo" dieting (when body weight goes up and down repeatedly) and other more severe dysfunctional eating patterns, such as anorexia nervosa, bulimia, and binge-eating disorders.

The word *diet* by itself can be confusing. We equate "going on a diet" with restricting our food intake in order to lose weight, but we also talk about eating a "balanced diet" when what we really mean is a meal plan. The "diets" that do not work in the long run are only the restrictive ones, not the balanced meal plans. In fact, meal planning is essential for the control and prevention of insulin resistance and diabetes, but "going on a diet" is a recipe for failure for the vast majority of people who do—young and old alike. Dieting is essentially an exercise in self-deprivation and food obsession. In order to follow any restrictive diet, you are forced to think about food all the time to remain constantly aware of which foods are "permitted" and which are "forbidden." However, it is human nature for a forbidden object to become an obsession; then we start craving it, and it becomes almost impossible to stop thinking about it, particularly if it is something pleasurable like certain foods.

All fad diets are potentially dangerous for growing kids, so first try adopting a reasonable meal plan, and weight loss will likely follow, although it may be slow. A painless way for any of your family members to lose a little weight is by following the 300/200 daily plan, a strategy that reinforces all of the lifestyle ideas incorporated into this book. Reflect on your current lifestyle with regard to your family's exercise and eating patterns. What would your kids be willing to change? Use these changes to reduce your family's caloric intake by just 300 calories a day, while adding in 200 calories' worth of physical activity daily. The net decrease of 500 calories per day, through a combination of eating a little less and moving a little bit more, can result in a one pound per week loss of fat weight (per person).

For example, to decrease calories by 300, simply replace your kids' sugared and other caloric drinks with low-calorie ones (you should implement this change anyway), have them eat healthier snacks like whole fruit in place of calorie-dense ones, and/or replace high-calorie condiments like mayonnaise and margarine with lower-calorie options. Simply taking slightly smaller portions at meals or leaving a few bites on your plate at each meal can also lower calorie intake. As for the 200 extra calories you want to expend, try taking a daily walk with your kids, have them walk the dog, take the stairs instead of the elevator, and/or add as many steps as possible to each day. Even the calories used when standing up and walking around for a few minutes after every 30 minutes of a sedentary activity will add up quickly.

Although you now know that weight loss alone is not mandatory for improved insulin action and diabetes control, studies have shown that a weight loss of just 11 pounds (5 kg) can, by itself, improve overall blood glucose control (measured by glucated hemoglobin) by 0.4 percent. A simple plan like the 300/200 one can assist with such a loss safely over just two to three months—and without making any radical lifestyle changes like most restrictive diets require!

PUTTING GOOD EATING INTO PRACTICE

WITH A FEW simple strategies, you can easily improve the nutritional quality of your family's diet. Some of these changes may appear obvious whereas others are strategies you may not have thought of before as being helpful. In any case, they are all fairly simple to include in your lifestyle. Tips for jump-starting your family into healthier eating are also included in this chapter.

General Tips for Eating More Healthfully

For starters, shop carefully and choose your selections wisely. If you simply choose not to buy certain foods, your kids will not be as likely to eat them, so only buy what you truly want your family to eat. It also helps to have fewer varieties of snack foods that you would prefer them to eat less of, such as cookies or chips. People tend to eat more when a larger selection is available, as they are more likely to take one of each of the different varieties in the pantry. If only one type of snack food is accessible, your kids may tire of it more quickly and look for other, more healthful types of foods to consume.

Keep in mind that your family will be more likely to consume enough of the key nutrients by eating a wide variety of wholesome, nutrient-rich foods, including colorful fruits and vegetables. Try to de-emphasize white potato products and iceberg lettuce as primary vegetables. French fries are loaded with more calories from fat than potato, and potatoes are a high-GI and -GL food, so do not consider french fries or potato chips a healthy substitute for other vegetables, particularly since potatoes are better considered a starch. Iceberg lettuce is largely made up of water with few other nutrients and very little fiber. White onions (another staple among kids) are reasonably heart healthy (containing lycopene, vitamin C, and potassium), but they are best eaten in forms other than deep-fat-fried, breaded onion rings! Likewise, it is okay for kids to eat processed tomatoes in the form of canned tomatoes or spaghetti sauce, but try to get them to use less ketchup and barbeque sauce, which are loaded with added sugar. For a healthier fare, try new potatoes (they have a lower GI than white ones), or better yet, sweet potatoes, along with Romaine or other dark green lettuces, spinach, and a wider variety of other nutrient-rich vegetables like broccoli, cauliflower, asparagus, and peppers instead.

Interestingly, not only what, but also how often you eat may affect your overall food intake as well as your risk of gaining extra fat pounds. Eating less at one sitting, but more frequently—which is how younger kids naturally eat—appears to be the best route to follow, regardless of your age. In one study, overweight men were found to consume fewer calories when presented with the same total amount of food divided up into several smaller meals instead of a single, larger one. In fact, people who are "grazers," eating lots of small meals and snacks throughout the day, are typically leaner than less frequently eating counterparts, even when eating equivalent calories. Thus, it appears that eating four to six smaller meals throughout the day may keep your metabolic rate at a higher level, thus increasing your overall energy expenditure for each day. An added benefit is that you probably will not become ravenously hungry between meals, which, by itself, may keep you from overeating.

The timing of meals, or skipping them altogether, also can affect your family's body weight and overall health. Surprisingly, that first meal of the day may be even more important for your kids than anyone ever realized. Breakfast eaters tend to be leaner than people who skip it, and skipping breakfast is actually associated with a greater risk of developing type 2 diabetes! More important, kids who eat breakfast are more likely to meet their growing bodies' daily needs for calcium, iron, and other essential nutrients.

More to the point, breakfast is one of the most important meals of the day because it serves to "break" your overnight fast, effectively kicking your fasting metabolism into a higher gear and lowering levels of hormones that increase insulin resistance. Conversely, skipping your first meal sustains your fasted state and keeps your body in a more economical "starvation" mode, which is energy conserving (meaning you expend fewer calories until you eat), and your body will likely remain less responsive to insulin during this time. So, make sure your kids break their fast by eating breakfast.

Also, one of the worst things you can do is to allow yourself to become overly hungry by skipping meals; doing so almost always results in overeating at later meals. People who eat most of their calories later in the day (7 P.M. or later) are generally more overweight as well, likely because eating larger amounts of food at one sitting leads to greater fat storage (your body can only use so many calories at one time). Excess calories in a given meal are stored as fat, which is done even more effectively in the evening when activity levels are generally lower. While sleeping, you experience your lowest level of energy expenditure of the day, which allows for optimum fat and energy storage. People who skip breakfast (and possibly lunch) and save their main calorie consumption for dinner invariably end up with higher levels of body fat for all of these reasons and have a greater risk of developing type 2 diabetes, despite having passed up a meal or two during the day.

Finally, select your foods carefully, paying close attention to the glycemic index and load of the foods that you purchase and consume. Eating nutritionally is a balancing act, whereby foods with a higher glycemic load can be balanced by limiting the total amount that you consume and by taking in more selections with a lower glycemic punch. Your family does not need to completely avoid all sugary or high-GI snacks, rather just limit your consumption of them. Instead of letting your youngsters fill up on nutrient-poor, high-calorie foods, balance their consumption of such items with an expanded intake of healthier snacks and meals with a higher satiety potential.

Tips for Cooking Healthier Meals

A lot of people may tell you that in order to prepare healthier meals and snacks for your family, you need to buy several new cookbooks for yourself—and doing so could get quite expensive! Unless you need some new ideas for meals, however, you can simply use and modify recipes from the cookbooks that you already have and still cook a healthier fare. Preparing more nutrient-dense, lower-calorie meals at home is easy to do by making small alterations to any recipes that you currently use. If you really want to try some new recipes, there is still no real need to spend more money; you can always take cookbooks out of the library or look online for recipe ideas.

For example, take a favorite family recipe, such as homemade macaroni and cheese. The ingredient list for one such recipe includes 1.5 cups of elbow macaroni, 3 tablespoons of butter, 2 cups of milk, 8 ounces sharp processed American cheese, ½ teaspoon salt, and pepper, as desired. The glycemic index and load table in the previous chap-

Summary of Simple Strategies
to Eat More Healthfully

•

- Pay careful attention to glycemic index and load when choosing foods
- Severely limit the quantity of "white" foods that your family consumes, including bread, rice, potatoes, sugar, and pasta
- Limit intake of any type of carbohydrate to no more than two servings: 1 cup cooked pasta, ⅔ cup rice, 2 slices of bread, and 3 ounces of potatoes
- Never let your kids eat more than one to two slices of pizza at a meal
- Balance glycemic load with greater intake of plenty of fiber-rich, lower-calorie foods (like vegetables) at meals (eaten first to induce early satiety)
- Always have your kids eat whole fruits rather than drinking fruit juices, and limit their intake of dried fruits to appropriate serving sizes
- Limit your family's intake of saturated and trans fats, replacing them with healthier fats, like monounsaturated
- Watch out for calorie-dense hidden fats in margarine, butter, mayonnaise, gravy, salad dressing, sour cream, cream, whole-milk products, and meat
- Watch out for excessive added sugars in many "low-fat" and "fat-free" foods
- Implement a fifteen-minute waiting period before allowing your kids to go back for second helpings, or better yet, just plan a light snack for two to three hours after eating
- Never make your kids feel obligated to finish all of the food on their plates, with the possible exception of their vegetables (if prepared without much added fat)
- Pack your own lunch and snacks for school, work, and everywhere else

- Avoid eating at buffet-style or all-you-can-eat restaurants, but if you do, limit your family to one plateful of salad and vegetables, followed by a smaller plateful of entrée items
- Allow your kids one small "treat" a day, but keep it moderate (equal to no more than 150 calories)
- Become an educated consumer and read food labels
- If you don't want your kids to eat as many nutrient-poor foods, then don't buy them (they may get them at school or from friends, but at least their access to such foods will be less)
- Keep fewer varieties of less healthy snacks (such as cookies or chips) on hand
- Minimize your consumption of all beverages containing added sugars, including soft drinks, Kool-Aid, Hi-C, Capri Sun, fruit "drinks," and sports drinks; try substituting flavored (noncaloric) or plain water instead.
- Never fall for food manufacturer's claims without reading food labels for yourself to identify added sugars and fats, and, of course, limit your consumption of them
- Limit your intake of highly processed foods and beverages, opting instead for more nutritious foods closer to their "natural" state
- Remember, "sugar-free" products are not necessarily sugar-free and are usually high in fat, "fat-free" ones are generally high in sugar, and neither are calorie-free
- Limit your intake of cholesterol, total fat (look for hidden fats), omega-6 fatty acids, and heart-unhealthy saturated or trans fats
- Colorize your dinner plates by trying to eat a wide variety of colored produce to obtain the key nutrients necessary for your kids' growth and good health
- Graze throughout the day rather than waiting until you are famished to eat
- Do not skip breakfast, as it increases your family's chances of gaining excess fat and developing type 2 diabetes

- Avoid eating large meals, especially later in the day, as doing so increases the likelihood that your family will store more fat
- Emphasize snacks, meals, and drinks with a lower glycemic index and load
- Increase your family's intake of fiber to recommended levels to increase satiety and decrease calorie consumption

ter lists macaroni in the "low GI, high GL" category, meaning that because of its high-fat content, it hits your bloodstream more slowly, even though its overall carbohydrate punch is significant. However, the butter, whole milk, and American cheese would make your meal high in fat—the saturated variety in particular—as well as calorie-dense.

How can you make this meal healthier without altering its flavor or making your kids turn up their noses at it? Actually, it's easy. First, consider buying some whole-wheat elbow macaroni to replace the regular type. For any pasta recipe, if your family balks at the heartier taste of the whole-wheat variety, try mixing the two types in equal amounts. As an alternative, read product labels carefully and choose a "reduced carb" pasta that contains extra fiber (and, thus, less digestible carbohydrate); while I would not recommend these as the only type of pasta you feed your kids, you could also mix this variety with traditional elbows to lower the carbohydrate content, if desired. For this recipe, also double the quantity of macaroni noodles to three cups (to lower the amount of cheesy sauce per serving).

Next, to reduce the saturated and trans fats and cholesterol from the butter, use margarine instead, specifically choosing one that is lower in these bad fats, such as Smart Balance. Similarly, use a lower-fat milk (2%, 1%, or skim), and substitute fat-free or 2% milk American cheese slices for the regular, fat-laden type. Finally, go easy on the salt, adding just enough for flavoring after the dish is cooked, which also allows you to add less overall. The end result of your changes will be a tasty, less caloric, and more nutrient-dense variety of a classic American meal. Its glycemic effects may be a little higher now with the reduced amount of fat, but you can easily compensate by eating a larger portion of veggies with your meal and a slightly smaller portion of macaroni and cheese.

You can make many other small changes in your family's recipes to improve their healthfulness and reduce their calorie content. Some of these improvements involve more careful shopping. For example, be aware that when a product states that it is a certain percentage of fat (e.g., 7 percent fat ground turkey), it refers to content of fat compared to the weight of the product, not its caloric contribution. Ground turkey that is 7 percent fat actually has over 8 grams of fat per serving, accounting for almost half of its calories; similarly, fat comprises a third of the calories in 2% milk and 17 percent of the total calories in the 1% variety.

If you are buying fat-free or reduced-fat products, keep in mind that many manufacturers replace the fat with added sugars, particularly in low-fat cookies and ice cream. As mentioned, the GI of such "treats" is often far higher than for the original, fat-filled variety, so instead buy the sugar-free variety of fat-reduced products (like ice cream) whenever possible, or stick with the original variety, but limit your family's intake.

As for fat, try to remove as much of it from foods as possible. In baked recipes, you can substitute applesauce or puréed prunes for the oil or fat to create a moist, virtually fat-free food. Substituting other ingredients, like two egg whites for each whole egg or plain yogurt or fat-free sour cream in place of regular sour cream, can also cut calories substantially without altering taste. Also, for the fats that you do use, choose heart-healthy fats like olive oil whenever possible. Healthy fats do not increase insulin resistance, and besides, they often increase satiety and lower the glycemic effects of the foods that they are found in. However, keep in mind that no matter what type of fat foods contain, fat still contains 100 calories per tablespoon.

Additional tips for healthier cooking and eating follow.

Specific Tips for Cooking Healthier Meals

•

- Cook with olive or canola oils, going easy on the oil (or using a cooking spray), and avoid frying foods
- Use lean cuts of meat, including beef with all visible fat removed, skinless chicken and turkey breast, lean ground beef, chicken or turkey, tofu, and soy protein
- Bake, broil, poach, or grill meat, fish, and chicken rather than frying them
- Buy lower-fat varieties of dairy products, including milk, cheese, sour cream, yogurt, and ice cream (combined with sugar-free whenever possible)
- Eat veggies raw, steamed, microwaved, or grilled, using only light seasonings rather than drenching them with creamy, cheesy, or buttery sauces
- Avoid cooking vegetables directly in water to prevent the loss of key vitamins and minerals into the liquid (or drink the "mineralized" water, too)
- Use mainly fresh or frozen vegetables and fruits as canned ones typically contain added salt and/or sugar, and only use canned fruit packed in natural juices
- Keep fresh vegetables such as baby carrots, broccoli, peppers, or cauliflower handy for snacks, and entice your kids to eat them with a healthy dip like hummus (chickpeas and sesame tahini) and fat-free or olive oil–based dressings
- Let your kids snack on whole fruits instead of manufactured products containing fruit, and keep a variety of fruits, such as grapes, apples, oranges, bananas, and seasonal fruit, on hand and in sight for healthy snacks
- If you drink fruit juices, use only the 100 percent juice varieties, and limit your consumption of those providing few nutrients, such as apple or white grape juice or any juice containing either of these two as a main ingredient

- On salads, use balsamic vinegar, reduced-calorie, or fat-free dressings, but still go easy on the amount that you use (keep in mind that dressings containing olive oil are still high in calories, while fat-free varieties often have added sugars)
- Add cut-up vegetables to canned beans, soups, or omelets to increase their nutrient value, water content, and general bulkiness
- Add extra whole-wheat pasta or brown rice to enhance pre-bought mixes like Rice-A-Roni or Chicken Helper containing only white versions of these starches; better yet, avoid prepackaged mixes, opting to season it yourself
- Buy only bread products that list whole wheat as the first ingredient on the food label, and use other whole-grain products whenever possible
- Add extra fiber into recipes for baked goods, casseroles, and soups by spooning in a few tablespoons of oat bran, wheat bran, or milled flaxseed during their preparation
- For baked goods, add only a half to two-thirds of the sugar that the recipe calls for and use healthier margarines instead of butter, shortening, or lard (or use the applesauce/puréed prune mixture)

Tips for Eating Out and Snacking on the Run

Have you ever walked into a convenience store feeling ravenous and tried to find a snack that was not full of sugar, fat, and/or salt? It is nearly impossible, with the possible exception of the selection of bottled water and diet drinks, not to mention the usually overripe bananas that some stores have available at the checkout counter! More often than not, though, finding healthy snacks and meals on the run is difficult at best.

Furthermore, portion sizes do count in eating nutritiously, and the ever-expanding portions of typical, ready-to-eat, popular foods contribute to the bulk of our caloric intake. How often have you or your kids grabbed a candy bar as a quick and easy snack? Maybe you consider yourself to be a bit more health-conscious, and you buy bagels or muffins for your family's snacking. Did you know that according to the serving sizes of the Food Guide Pyramid, a bagel counts for two servings, and most ready-to-eat muffins equal four? A package of cookies may contain up to eight times the amount of a single serving, a typical steak three times, cooked pasta six times, and most sodas twice as much.

Eating Restaurant Meals

Eating nutritiously in a restaurant—particularly a fast-food one—can be equally challenging. In fact, people who eat out at restaurants frequently are more overweight than those who make a habit out of eating home-cooked meals, and as a nation, we now eat out one meal in three (as compared with one out of twenty three decades ago). Fast-food fares generally consist of high-fat, high-GI, calorie-dense, and nutrient-poor choices, and food eaten in more formal dining settings (sit-down restaurants) is typically higher in fat than home-cooked versions.

In spite of all of our labor-saving devices, life for most people occurs at a more hectic pace nowadays—whether we are working long hours, taking the kids to a million different activities, or passing time stuck in traffic. As a result, more of us eat on the run, and eating out makes us fatter because, on the whole, restaurant portions are huge! Portion sizes at restaurants have been increasing steadily over the past several decades, with super-sized "value" menus plentiful and inexpensive.

In addition, buffet-style meals are abundant in pizza, Chinese, steakhouse, and other restaurants. (Remember what was mentioned earlier about how people eat more when their choices are more abundant or varied? Having a wide variety of fruits and vegetables to choose from, however, should be encouraged.) Invariably, people eat more than they need when exposed to an all-you-can-eat situation. Sit-down restaurant serving sizes have also steadily increased over the past several decades, and many studies show that when people are given larger portions, they eat more (and, thus, more calories) than if they had a smaller portion.

In my opinion, the biggest problem with eating out, particularly in most fast-food restaurants, is that it is difficult or impossible to feel satiated without overloading on calories. The portions given are too large, and the fat content is higher than in home-cooked foods. Also, it is very difficult to get enough vegetables, salad, or fresh fruit, particularly selections that have not been doctored with extra fat calories in the form of butter, oil, dressing, or whipped cream. As discussed, meals with a high glycemic index may end up making you feel hungrier in the long run than lower-GI ones, even though you have eaten an adequate (or possibly excessive) number of calories.

Personally, I first noticed this phenomenon almost a decade ago when I used to take my then young sons to McDonald's (one with a play place, of course!) for a "Happy Meal" comprised of four chicken nuggets and french fries. After finishing their meals, they would, unbelievably, still be clamoring for more food even though I knew that they had eaten more than enough calories for their small bodies. To deal with this problem, I started bringing a bag of baby carrots with us whenever we went out to eat, along with an apple or two. The very few additional calories they took in with these high-fiber "treats" filled them up completely, much better than an ice cream sundae (which we mistakenly tried on one occasion). This experience just reiterates the fact that what fast-food restaurants really need to offer their customers is a greater selection of fruits and vegetables. Of note, McDonald's has apparently recently added some fruit to their kids' meals, as has Wendy's.

The Center for Science in the Public Interest (CSPI) picked the best and the worst American fast foods in 2002, concluding that fast-food menus are getting better and worse at the same time, although many major fast-food chains appear to be responding to consumer demands for healthier options. On the better side were two items offered at Burger King and one each at McDonald's, Wendy's, and Subway. Completely

Center for Science in the Public Interest's Best and Worst Fast Food Fare (2002)

•

Best Fare: Wendy's mandarin chicken salad (only use half the packet of dressing, though); Burger King's Chicken Whopper Jr. (but do not order the more caloric regular version); Subway's low-fat subs ("7 subs with 6 grams of fat or less," including honey mustard ham, sweet onion chicken teriyaki, and red wine vinaigrette club sandwiches); McDonald's fruit 'n yogurt parfait (containing only 2 grams of saturated fat and ⅔ cup of berries); and Burger King's BK veggie burger.

Worst Fare: Burger King's old-fashioned ice cream shake (clocking in with almost 800 calories for the medium, 1,200 for the large version, and loaded with saturated and trans fats, it is worse for your heart than even the worst burgers); french fries (a king size order has 600 calories and 30 grams of fat, half of them heart unhealthy); hash browns (15 grams of saturated plus trans fats in the large order); Double Whopper with cheese (with more calories than any other burger because of its wider bun and double layer of burgers, this gem has 1,150 calories and 33 grams of saturated/trans fat); and, finally, its value meals (such meals' caloric values range from 1,300 to 2,100, a full day's calories for many adults).

sweeping the worst category, however, was also Burger King, although many other fast-food servers undoubtedly deserve to share the honor.

In a surprise move, McDonald's recently did away with its "supersize" menu, thus cutting out its super-sized (7 ounces) french fries and 42-ounce drinks. While the thought is good, in reality, getting the 6-ounce "large" fries instead of the former super-sized option only saves a small number of calories (less than 100 calories and 4 grams of fat).

However, any food modifications that involve little changes in our behavior as consumers may be promising. Fat reduction is an easy approach to reducing the calorie content of foods without changing the portion size, but simply reducing their overall energy density is likely a better solution, which can be accomplished by increasing their water content with the addition of more vegetables, fruits, and whole grains. Doing so would allow consumers to eat their usual portions while taking in fewer calories.

It is not likely that all fast-food restaurants are going to do away with their value menus anytime soon, though, so we desperately need to teach our kids how to be more educated about what they are eating. The trend nowadays is for people to think that the carbohydrate, protein, and fat content (e.g., the low-carb craze) is what is most important to pay attention to, when in reality, appropriate portions and the energy density of foods is infinitely more relevant. By the time kids reach the age of five, they show a more adult response to portion sizes, eating more when the portions increase. Thus, we still need to teach our kids that eating huge portions of energy-dense foods (and, thus, excess calories) will have a negative effect on their health and that they can have better health simply by filling up instead on larger portions of foods lower in energy density, such as fruits and vegetables, which are still difficult to get enough of on most fast-food menus.

Eating School Lunches

Maybe you already carefully regulate what your family eats at home or in restaurants, but what about at school? Think your children are being served a healthy fare with school lunches? You may want to think again!

Yes, the federal government mandates what constitutes a nutritious lunch for our kids, but their requirements far from guarantee that it is actually nutritious; on the contrary, public school lunches are notoriously high in fat and calories. Keep in mind that the school breakfast and lunch programs were begun only to ensure that all children received "adequate" nutrition—defined as at least two-thirds of their recommended daily calorie intake—so that low-income students were not missing meals and negatively affecting their ability to learn. To subsidize the plan, every year, the USDA buys millions of pounds of excess beef, pork, milk, and other meat and dairy products to bolster sagging prices in the livestock industry. These high-fat, high-cholesterol products are then distributed at very low cost to the national school lunch program. When the program was begun, though, kids were more physically active than they currently are, not to mention that nowadays, even low-income kids usually have access to inexpensive (but not necessarily nutritious) food.

To top it off, many cash-strapped schools have also brought in private fast-food vendors, such as Taco Bell and Pizza Hut, allowing them to sell their food to your kids for lunch at a reasonable price (even in elementary schools). Why would schools knowingly subject their students to such low-nutrition food? The reason is simple, really: economics. The schools, many of which are now severely underfunded at the federal, state, and local levels, receive 50 percent of the money from the sales of such food—but at the expense of our children's health.

In addition, haven't you ever noticed the ubiquitous, brightly colored, and appealing soft drink and other vending machines placed in your child's school? Soft drinks are a relatively inexpensive source of calories, increasing in price with inflation relatively less than milk or bottled water, and schools again get a cut of all vending machine profits. It will come as no surprise to you that a nationwide survey of vending machines in middle and high schools recently revealed that 75 percent of the drinks and 85 percent of the snacks sold are of poor nutritional value.

Some public school administrators are finally beginning to fight back, though. Los Angeles and Oakland public schools imposed a ban on the sale of soft drinks in cafeterias and vending machines in all of their schools. The new policy is to substitute bottled water, milk, fruit drinks with at least 50 percent fruit juice, and sports drinks with less than 42 grams of sugar per 20-ounce serving (the same amount of added sugar that a typical 12-ounce soft drink contains). Containing 20 grams of sugar, 12 ounces of Gatorade or other sports drink still typically has a dramatic effect on glycemia, but this amount is, nevertheless, about 20 fewer grams of carbohydrates than a typical can of sugared soda. In addition, the state of Texas bans the sale of all junk food on its public school campuses during lunchtime.

Eating more nutritiously at school may have a greater effect than previously thought. The "Peak Performance Program" in schools throughout Illinois, Indiana, Wisconsin, and Minnesota, which had initiated the removal of candy and soft drink machines from schools and their replacement with readily available fruits, vegetables, whole grains, and energy drinks to combat childhood obesity, also recorded dramatic improvements in student learning and behavior as an added benefit. If you currently live in a state without such improvements in place, you can still band together with other concerned parents and contact your schools' administrators about initiating similar policies where you live.

You may be wondering how different it really is for your kids to bring their own lunches to school. On average, home-packed bag lunches contain 21 grams of fat per meal, the recommended amount for lunch for middle schoolers, compared with 31 grams in typical school lunches—a 10-gram difference that equates to 90 calories. Furthermore, à la carte items such as pizza, baked goods, chips, and candy sold at schools also contribute to excessive fat consumption by students.

To reduce fat intake, schools need to introduce lower-fat versions of popular foods as well as reduce the cost and variety of low-fat items. Some schools have indeed been moving in this direction: In 2003, the Physicians' Committee for Responsible Medicine (PCRM) reported that the "most improved player" award belonged to the Detroit City School District, which made menu changes that included daily offerings of fruits and vegetables, calcium-fortified juices, meatless entrées, and whole-grain breads, as well as vegan burgers three times per week. The district is still also investigating the possibility of offering calcium-fortified soy milk and more soy-based and legume-based entrées for the lunch menu.

Other such interventions have been successful in several elementary schools around the country where energy intake from fat fell by 7 percent in improved lunches, accomplished together with another positive health improvement: the implementation of more moderate- to vigorous-intensity physical activities for schoolchildren. Careful attention will need to be paid, however, to ensure that the fat removed from school lunches is not simply replaced with added sugars and refined products with a large glycemic effect, or the healthiness of the lunches will not have been improved at all for prediabetic or diabetic kids!

A recent study showed that when lower-fat interventions were implemented for school lunches in select schools in New England, the content of added sugars in the lunches did indeed increase, mainly due to the inclusion of items such as fruit juices and chocolate milk. The specific need of diabetic kids for such a nutritional balancing act makes it all the more important to emphasize the substitution of fats with high-fiber, lower-GI carbohydrate alternatives rather than foods high in added sugars, or the result may be that your child's blood sugars may rise even more from these so-called "healthier" lunches.

Admittedly, it is more arduous for time-pressed parents and their kids to worry about packing a lunch and snacks for kids to take to school everyday than to shell out money to buy an already prepared lunch, but it is well worth the effort to pack your own, and it is really not that difficult. First, start with a lower glycemic carbohydrate, such as whole-wheat bread or a pita pocket. Then, make sure to include some protein as it takes longer to metabolize, has little effect on glycemia, keeps kids more alert, and increases satiety. Some good sources are sliced, lean meats (e.g., turkey breast), cheese (part skim, low-fat, or fat-free), light yogurt, peanut butter, hard-boiled eggs, tuna, and hummus. Balance it out with some easy-to-eat vegetables, like carrot sticks or cucumber slices, and some fresh or dried fruit (cut into small pieces for easier consumption, if needed). Adding in a less nutritious snack or dessert like potato chips, pretzels, a granola bar, or a small cookie is certainly allowed (assuming your child eats the healthier items); even if some of these items have a

Specific Tips for Eating Out or on the Run

•

- Try to eat out less often since it is harder to get foods that are nutrient-dense, but not high-calorie, unless you fix them yourself
- Seek out healthier selections on any fast-food or other restaurant menu, including items with a lower saturated fat, sugar, and calorie content
- When you do eat out, be more conscious about portion sizes; take home part of your meal in a "doggie bag," and avoid all-you-can-eat restaurants
- Never "super-size" your meal; in fact, go for the junior-size options whenever possible instead (particularly when it comes to french fries)
- Order a salad to accompany your meal, or if you prefer, bring a bag of fresh veggies or a piece of fresh fruit along to eat
- If you order a salad out, always ask for the dressing on the side so that you can add it yourself (and then do so sparingly, regardless of the fat content); do the same with other calorie-dense toppings like sour cream, cheese, and bacon
- For other items like potatoes, order the butter and all other sauces on the side so that you can control how much you consume
- Skip the sugared soft drink and their noncarbonated, sugar-filled cousins, replacing them with a diet soft drink (a noncaffeinated, non-cola variety), water, or skim milk
- Whenever possible, have your kids bring their own lunch to school to ensure that their meal is lower in fat and higher in fiber and nutrition
- Pack snacks for your kids that have less added sugar and a lower glycemic index and load, such as fruit, vegetables, reduced-fat cheeses, nuts, or light yogurt

higher GI, the lower GI of the rest of the meal will lower the glycemic effect somewhat. Finally, throw in a healthy beverage (plain bottled or calorie-free flavored water, low-fat milk, or a caffeine-free diet soft drink), and your child will have a nutritionally balanced, healthy lunch everyday—instead of a fat- and sugar-laden one that may negatively raise blood sugars and affect his or her ability to concentrate on schoolwork.

An added tip to make your mornings flow more smoothly is to plan ahead and pack most or all of your children's lunches the night before. Also, if you are fresh out of ideas when it comes to appetizing yet healthy lunches to pack for your kids, check around for good books and articles on the topic. One I would particularly recommend, *American Dietetic Association Guide to Healthy Eating for Kids,* particularly focuses on kids in the five- to twelve-year-old range and contains an entire chapter on creating nutritious bag lunches for your kids.

Tips for Jump-starting Your Family's Healthier Eating Plan

Are you still not convinced that you can actually get your kids to eat healthier foods if you buy them? Most parents know that their children should be eating better, but more times than not, they let their kids eat the less healthy selections because when parents try substituting healthier alternatives for junk food, their kids turn up their noses at the new selection. In addition to following the tips for cooking and eating more healthfully given in this chapter, here are some additional ideas about what frustrated parents can do to more easily get their kids "with the program."

You may also still be unsure of what would qualify as a healthier alternate. Unfortunately, current marketing practices have made it difficult for the average consumer to easily tell, particularly when controlling blood sugars is a concern. If you believe everything that you hear, you may think that switching your children to snacking on yogurt and granola bars is the healthiest way to go, but you would be wrong—at

Suggestions for Making a Smoother Transition to Healthier Eating

•

- Make small changes in your shopping habits rather than eliminating junk food all at once; going "cold turkey" will be too hard on everyone in the family
- Have healthy snacks in plain view in the refrigerator and cupboards; if your kids can see them, they are more likely to eat them
- Keep a variety of healthy choices on hand as your kids are more likely to get bored with limited, healthier choices
- Rather than eliminating dessert (if you usually serve one), simply substitute healthier choices, like low-fat yogurt, reduced-fat/reduced-sugar ice cream, or fruit
- Always let your kids eat when they are truly hungry, but teach them the difference between physical hunger and eating out of boredom
- Talk to your kids about how you are changing what you are eating to get healthy, rather than talking about losing weight or dieting
- Become the portion police: Allocate snacks in more appropriate amounts and put your kids' food on their plates for them at meals
- Never use food as a reward or as a means to soothe your kids' emotional upset

least partially. For instance, many varieties of yogurt contain as much fat and sugar as regular ice cream and would, therefore, be no better for your kids to eat. Similarly, most granola bars are high in carbohydrates and fat, and even most rice cakes nowadays have so much added sugar that they have an extremely high glycemic effect.

Although there are undoubtedly many appropriate snacks that you can try that your kids will like, see page 91 for a list of some healthy (and

Healthier Snacks Your Kids Will Like
(I Promise!)

•

- Raw veggies (carrots, cucumbers, cauliflower, etc.), plus up to 2 tablespoons of fat-free ranch or honey Dijon dressing, or hummus
- A piece of fresh fruit (or 1 cup of fruit)
- A small handful of pretzels (1 ounce or less) with a similar serving of peanuts (or other nuts)
- One low-sugar rice cake with peanut butter (no more than 2 tablespoons)
- 5 to 6 whole-grain crackers (1 ounce), plus peanut butter or 1 ounce of low-fat cheese
- One moderate handful of nuts or seeds (1 ounce or less)
- 3 to 4 cups of low-fat microwave or air-popped popcorn without added butter
- Reduced calorie (low-fat, sugar-free) yogurt, with or without ½ of a sliced banana
- 1 ounce of low-fat or fat-free cheese (or one stick of part-skim string cheese)
- Low-fat frozen yogurt bar or frozen fruit bar (choose ones with total carbs less than 15 to 20 grams)
- Sugar-free Popsicle
- Sugar-free Jell-O, with or without added canned fruit (packed in its own juices)
- 1 to 2 ounces lean or fat-free lunch meat (turkey breast, for example)
- 1 hard-boiled egg with yolk, or whites only from 3 to 4 hard-boiled eggs
- 1 medium dill pickle (high sodium content, though)
- 1 cup broth-based vegetable soup (Watch sodium content, though. Look for Healthy Choice soups or other products with a low sodium content.)

diabetes savvy) snack ideas to use as a starting place. If controlling portion sizes is a problem (e.g., your kids help themselves to these snacks while you are not at home), try buying single-serving-size packets of these items when applicable (like for pretzels) until an appropriate portion becomes more second nature to them. You may also want to invest in a small kitchen scale that can be used to weigh out ounces of food; you will likely be amazed at how much you have been overestimating the actual size of most servings.

If eaten in the recommended portions, the listed snacks should have a minimal effect on blood glucose levels. For teens, two selections from the list may be needed to satisfy hunger. If this is the case, try to combine a carbohydrate-based choice with one that contains fewer grams of carbohydrate to keep the snack from causing an excessive rise in blood sugars. Of course, this list is by no means exhaustive. Be inventive and come up with other fun snacks that your kids appreciate simply by keeping in mind that it's always best to avoid low-nutrition "white" foods, added sugars, saturated and trans fats, and large portions of foods with a higher glycemic effect. Additionally, kids can always eat any of the "free foods" included in the diabetes exchange diet (listed in appendix B).

Paying attention to your family's eating is essential to controlling obesity and preventing diabetes, but we have yet to discuss another equally if not more important lifestyle habit: physical activity. In the next couple of chapters, the importance of being physically active is covered. Before you read on, though, stand up, stretch, and walk around for a few minutes. (After you read the next chapters, you will truly understand why I asked you to.) In the next chapter, you will learn more about how physical activity can help keep blood sugars in check.

EXERCISE FOR PREVENTING AND CONTROLLING TYPE 2 DIABETES

T HERE IS no doubt that exercise is good for everyone, young and old alike. Being physically active improves the function of your heart and your cardiovascular system as well as the endurance, tone, and size of your muscles. You may feel tired exercising, but overall it increases your energy level rather than decreasing it. Being physically active on a regular basis is also associated with better self-esteem, an improved body image, reduction in anxiety and depression, and other psychological perks. The best part about exercise, though, is that it uses up energy and keeps you from storing as many excess calories as fat.

Researchers have found a clear association between physical inactivity and childhood obesity—and overweight adults for that matter. The presence of this recent epidemic in our youth is essentially a symptom of the unhealthy behaviors and lifestyles that plague our society. Children in the United States today spend, on average, five to six hours a day involved in sedentary pursuits during their leisure time, including television watching, playing video games, and using computers. If they were sufficiently active during the day at school, such sedentary pursuits might not matter as much, but unfortunately, our kids are not physically active enough at school to make up for their inactivity at home and at other times.

You may be wondering exactly how much of a contribution a sedentary lifestyle is actually making to the dual epidemics of obesity and type 2 diabetes in America's youth. If our children were to start exercising more, would being active be enough to prevent or rid them of both conditions? If they are more fit, but still overweight, do their bodies benefit as much from the physical activity? The answers to these questions and more will be addressed in this chapter.

Adults are notorious for regaining lost weight after a diet ends, and children are no different. As for elevated blood sugars, perhaps with regular exercise and some dietary improvements, your child's blood sugars may become normal, despite his or her "at-risk" or diagnosed status, but technically, once someone has been diagnosed with diabetes, it is never considered to be totally gone even if blood sugars normalize. Unfortunately, if you ever revert to the same lifestyle habits that contributed to its development in the first place, it almost assuredly will "return." The same can be said about a state of insulin resistance, or prediabetes. However, mounting evidence indicates that exercise may be effective in preventing type 2 diabetes from manifesting in the first place and in helping to control it in people with the condition.

Exercise to Reduce Diabetes Risk

Over the past decade, many studies have assessed people's exercise habits and concluded that regular physical activity is associated with a lower risk for the development of type 2 diabetes. However, much of this research was done with cross-sectional studies—that is, looking at large numbers of people after the fact using questionnaires or brief physical exams to assess their current health status, lifestyle habits, and risk— and heavily relied on often unreliable, self-reported exercise habits. Nevertheless, "active" individuals were generally reported to be leaner, with lower levels of abdominal fat, better glucose levels and insulin action, and a lower risk of developing diabetes than their sedentary counterparts.

Only recently have several landmark research studies *directly* assessed the impact of regular physical activity on the prevention of type 2 diabetes. The Diabetes Prevention Program (DPP) did just that when it studied 3,234 overweight American adults with impaired glucose tolerance at high risk for diabetes. Of the participants, at least 45 percent were African-Americans or Hispanics, populations known for having the highest risk of developing it. The adults in the "lifestyle arm" of the study were asked to follow a low-fat diet and increase their exercise to include 150 minutes (2.5 hours) per week of a moderate-intensity activity like brisk walking, spread out over at least three days and done for a minimum of ten minutes at a time. After three years, these participants had lowered their average risk of developing diabetes by a whopping 58 percent, despite their high risk status. Moreover, this reduced risk was evident regardless of their ethnicity, age, or sex—in fact, the effect was even greater among older individuals.

Since the DPP study utilized combined lifestyle changes, it did not directly test the contribution of physical activity alone, without concomitant changes in diet and body weight. The active DPP participants lost an average of 7 percent of their body weight, which would amount to only a loss of 14 pounds in a 200-pound person. A study in Finland found a similar reduction in the risk for diabetes after their participants lost body weight, lowered their fat intake, ate less saturated fat and more fiber, and added thirty minutes of daily walking and occasional resistance training to their regimens. While simultaneous changes in both diet and exercise habits are undoubtedly the best way to prevent or control diabetes, the contribution of exercise by itself is believed by many to be the more crucial of the two.

When you start to exercise, your body immediately responds by releasing "stress" hormones that work to increase your blood sugar. Humans have a limited supply of glucose stored in their muscles and liver (glycogen) and even less circulating in the bloodstream. Blood sugar levels must be maintained for your brain and nervous system to function properly. Thus, since carbohydrates are the primary fuel that the body uses during any exercise, your liver must act quickly to replace the blood sugar muscles use by breaking down its glycogen to form glucose or making new glucose from metabolic precursors like lactic acid. These stress hormones signal the liver to begin releasing more glucose; a pancreatic hormone called glucagon is the one with the most direct effect on that organ. Epinephrine (adrenaline) raises your heart rate and signals your exercising muscles to break down their stored glycogen and some fat as well. At the same time, your body reduces the amount of insulin the pancreas secretes, which helps to keep the muscles from taking up too much blood glucose. Other hormones, such as norepinephrine, growth hormone, and cortisol, effectively redistribute more blood and provide other fuels to working muscles and the liver.

While stress hormones are generally effective in maintaining blood sugars during exercise, there may be times when your family's glucose levels are already higher than normal, such as after eating a meal with a high GI and/or GL. In this instance, you would like exercise to help lower your sugar level, not simply maintain it. The bad news, though, is that exercise can raise, maintain, or lower blood sugar levels, depending on what you choose to do for your activity: How fast you move, how hard you work out, and how long you are active can all affect the energy needs of working muscles and can differently influence blood sugars as well. For example, many endurance athletes develop hypoglycemia (low blood sugar) at the end of a marathon-length run or workout due to the extreme demands that extended, higher-intensity activities put on the body's carbohydrate stores. On the other hand, heavy weight lifting (involving hard bursts of activity done for only a short time) can actually cause stress hormones to produce more blood glucose than your body needs, causing blood sugars to rise temporarily.

The best way to anticipate your body's blood sugar response to exercise is to understand which of your three energy systems predominates for a specific activity done for a given length of time. Regardless of the system used to supply energy, all muscular contractions are fueled directly by a substance known as ATP (adenosine triphosphate). For short, powerful, anaerobic activities like sprinting or heavy weight lifting, the first energy system, the phosphagens (stored ATP and creatine phosphate), make ATP rapidly available to muscles; however, this system will only provide energy for up to ten seconds of all-out activity. Once it begins to lose its ATP-making capacity, the lactic acid system, our second system, gears up and provides additional energy for up to about two minutes. Neither one of these systems uses oxygen (making them "anaerobic"), and both make relatively little ATP, but their use actually slightly raises blood sugars temporarily due to the heightened release of stress hormones that accompanies them.

Prepubescent kids are best suited for phosphagen use, meaning that they are good at doing short, intense bouts of activity. Haven't you ever noticed how when you take a walk with a small child, he or she wants to run ahead and then wait for you to catch up (you know, the tortoise and the hare scenario)? Kids are naturally doing what their bodies are best suited to do. Before reaching puberty, however, kids are much less efficient at using the second (lactic acid) system, so for this and other reasons—including their immature bones, muscles, and nerves—heavy weight lifting is definitely not recommended for prepubescent children, although mild to moderate training is allowed.

The third and final energy system, the aerobic or oxygen system, fuels all activities that use the major muscle groups and are sustained for two minutes or longer by making large quantities of ATP oxidatively (meaning by using oxygen), but at a slower rate than by other means.

Your muscles must have access to a steady supply of ATP during prolonged activities, such as walking, running, cycling, and swimming. The fuels supplying this system are any of the macronutrients stored in various depots around your body—carbohydrates in muscles, liver, and blood; fats in adipose and muscle; and proteins in muscles—making it the most versatile of the three systems. When you are resting, your body usually uses a mix of about 60 percent fat and 40 percent carbohydrate (with insignificant protein use). During exercise, carbohydrates supply the majority of the fuel, even more so when you work out harder. Fat can also be used, but contributes most during mild to moderate workouts. During recovery from exercise, though, when your body is restocking fuel depots that were used, fat use again predominates. Luckily, prepubescent youth are able to increase the capacity of their aerobic systems to almost the same extent as teens and adults simply by participating regularly in such activities.

So, why would anyone want to exercise intensely if it raises blood sugar levels? One reason is that the effect is temporary: Blood sugars will usually return back to normal within an hour. A more relevant consideration is the fact that almost any exercise may enhance insulin sensitivity and glucose tolerance for a period of time afterward, making physical activity of utmost importance to diabetes prevention and control. Both recent exercise and regular exercise training appear to have favorable effects on blood glucose and insulin action in almost everyone. For starters, when carbohydrate use is significant, as it is during thirty minutes of continuous, moderate exercise, blood sugar levels in people with diabetes usually decrease during the activity. Then, for two or more hours afterward, the prior exercise causes an enhanced uptake of blood sugar *without insulin*. In fact, a single workout—particularly if prolonged or intense—can enhance insulin action for twenty-four hours or more while glycogen stores in muscles and the liver are being replenished.

Regular exercise also increases your muscles' overall sensitivity to insulin, allowing for more effective blood glucose use and control. Having a greater muscle mass as a result of training also enhances this effect. It is well known that physically trained people have a heightened sensitivity to insulin, but training-induced improvements in insulin-resistant or diabetic individuals are often even more pronounced. A recent lifestyle intervention study involving sedentary, insulin-resistant, middle-aged adults showed that thirty minutes of moderate walking, done three to seven days per week for six months, succeeded in reversing their prediabetic state—without a change in their diets or any loss of body weight. Similar improvements in glucose tolerance have been found in older adults (average age of seventy-two years) who engaged in low- to moderate-intensity "walking" on mini-trampolines for twenty to forty minutes four days per week over a four-month period. Enhanced glucose uptake was seen among these participants without any additional insulin release or loss of abdominal fat.

Unfortunately, results from adult studies cannot be directly applied to our youth since their metabolisms differ, and fewer studies have been done on kids alone. However, it is known that exercise training can improve the action of insulin in obese people of *all* ages within just one week of training, suggesting that insulin sensitivity can be acutely enhanced without weight loss and without evoking a true training adaptation in muscle. Moreover, a study conducted on lean but sedentary young adult women (ages eighteen to thirty-five) undertaking either six months of thrice-weekly aerobic or resistance (weight) training showed that either form of training improves glucose use, although by different mechanisms. Weight training resulted in more muscle mass, allowing for greater overall glucose uptake. While endurance (aerobic) training did not change their amount of muscle as much, it did increase their muscular capacity to use glucose, again without changes in body weight or abdominal fat. So, both aerobic and anaerobic training will improve sensitivity to insulin and, as a result, lower any elevations in blood glucose levels.

Thus, it appears that any type of exercise makes insulin work better in adults and kids alike. When less insulin is needed, your pancreas is more likely to be able to produce enough insulin to meet your body's needs, and blood glucose levels or your risk for developing type 2 diabetes will vastly decrease, even without a change in body weight. If better insulin action due to exercise is not a potential "cure" for diabetes, then I really have no idea what is.

Physical Activity and Weight Loss

Exactly why is expending extra energy through exercise so important, especially for our youth? For starters, the obesity epidemic shows no signs of abating, and as a society, we have an urgent need to fight back against this progressive overweight state before it's too late. Surprisingly, despite the hundreds of thousands of calories—even millions for some—that we eat in the course of a year, we can maintain our body weight within a pound or two, which demonstrates the innate aptitude of the human body to tightly regulate food intake to match calorie use. Despite this ability, more people than ever before in our history—adults, teenagers, and children alike—are gradually becoming overfat instead, primarily because they are not expending enough calories through physically activity.

Weight gain is usually subtle, resulting in "creeping obesity," which comes on slowly and steadily over a few years a little bit at a time. Since this weight is not being gained overnight, it is not too late to prevent or reverse this trend. For example, if your child eats just *50 calories* a day more than he or she expends (equal to only half a can of regular soda, a small apple, or about five or six peanut M&M's), the total weight gained in a year from that small excess is *five pounds* of body fat (a pound of fat equals 3,500 calories). Alternately, what if your child expends an extra 50 calories a day by adding in little bits of exercise throughout the day—easily accomplished with some extra walking, stretching, or other mild activity? Then the weight gain from these extra calories is totally avoided. Moreover, using exercise to expend an extra 50 calories a day beyond caloric needs results in a net *loss* of five pounds in a year for your child.

Using data from national surveys, some researchers assert that it will likely take an extra expenditure more in the range of 100 calories per day (from reduced food intake and increased physical activity combined) to prevent weight gain in most of the population, which could be easily achieved by small changes in behavior, such as adding in fifteen minutes of walking per day or eating a few less bites at each meal. In school-age children, it may be accomplished with a permanent reduction in the time spent on "screen" activities, such as TV watching and computer use, to achieve this difference. The bottom line, though, is that being physically active (especially with modern-day calorie intakes) makes a big difference in whether your family will experience overall weight gain, maintenance, or loss.

When I hear that someone is physically inactive, two almost inevitable health problems looming over that person immediately come to mind: an insulin-resistant state and fat weight gain. Just recently, a study showed that a poor diet and inactivity together were poised to overtake smoking as the leading cause of preventable death. You now know about the positive impact exercise has on insulin action; in short, the best way to prevent insulin resistance and type 2 diabetes is by exercising regularly. As for how to prevent excess weight gain, the answer is exactly the same.

Have you or your kids ever lost weight only to find that you could never maintain the weight loss? If so, you are not alone. An estimated 95 percent of dieters lose weight only to regain the same amount (or more) within six months to a year. In addition, most Americans have very little success in preventing weight gain with aging. Does this mean that your family should give up trying, that you are undeniably doomed to suffer from being overfat and out of shape? No, absolutely not! The solution is simply to get active and stop worrying so much about losing a certain amount of weight.

Even if you can't lose all the weight you desire, you can achieve a higher level of fitness, and doing so will undeniably benefit your health. Over the years, research has examined the effects of being fat and/or fit, separately and combined, on the risk of developing a debilitating illness or dying. The main finding has been that as your BMI increases, so does your risk of dying from heart disease. On a more positive note, the more physically fit you are, the lower your risk of dying for any reason becomes.

A recent study specifically addressed the issues of fatness versus fitness—at least in adults—and showed that both increased fatness and unfitness are independent risk factors for dying. Healthwise, the best scenario is to be "fit and thin." Although being fit cannot completely reverse the elevated risks arising from excess body fat, being classified as "fit and fat" appears to at least put you on a level playing field with people who are thin but unfit. The worst thing to be, indisputably, is a member of the "unfit and fat" club. In other words, although being overly fat is not ideal for your family's health, the overall metabolic effect of excess body fat can at least be favorably moderated by regular physical activity.

Why is being sedentary so damaging to your body? Basically, the wonderful, insulin-sensitizing effects of acute exercise and exercise training mentioned previously are transient—they do not last long after you revert to a sedentary state. In fact, while the effects of a single workout may last from an hour (following short, mild exercise) up to a day or two (for prolonged, intense activities), the effects of regular training begin to reverse within two to three days. Granted, if you have increased your muscle mass with training, all of your gains will not be lost in that short period of time, but with continued inactivity, they certainly will. Unfortunately, the saying, "If you don't use it, you lose it," definitely applies to training-induced enhancements in insulin action and glucose tolerance, as well as to all of exercise's other health benefits.

An added benefit of exercise is that even if it does not make you lose all of the weight you desire, it can still prevent you from gaining any more and positively modify your body composition (that is, cause you to lose fat while you gain muscle, which may keep your weight from changing much). Although diets are not generally recommended for youth, many adults report trying to lose or maintain their body weight by dieting, yet very few are also using exercise to aid them. To me, this makes absolutely no sense. These dieters must be avoiding exercise either out of ignorance or because they have yet to really believe how important it is in weight control.

A landmark study set out to prove what it takes to be successful in maintenance of lost body weight, and their results confirm what I personally knew all along: Exercise matters! Over the past decade, a national weight control registry has tracked individuals who have lost at least thirty pounds *and* kept the weight off for at least a year. Although that may not sound that difficult, keeping lost weight off for a year is actually not common at all among dieters; in reality, most people who lose weight gain it all back within six months. Although "members" of the registry have used a variety of weight-loss plans or methods (from a typical lower-calorie, moderate-carbohydrate diet like Weight Watchers to the famed low-carb Atkins diet), almost all of them share two lifestyle habits to keep the weight off: They continue to be conscientious about what they eat (eating more healthful food in appropriate portions), and they exercise almost daily, expending about 2,000 calories a week in physical activity. So, if your family wants to maintain any weight losses, get yourselves up off the couch and go for a walk (and do it again tomorrow, and the next day, and the next, and so on).

Diabetes and Physical Activity

Have you ever heard the expression, "Laughter is the best medicine"? For me, it always conjures up images of a Gary Larson cartoon where a group of medical doctors are depicted standing around a hospitalized patient in his bed, with all of the doctors pointing their fingers at him and laughing. Unfortunately, in that scenario, the doctors are the only ones experiencing the mentally soothing effects of beta-endorphin release.

Similarly, exercise as the best medicine should not be thought of as merely consisting of watching sporting events; on the contrary, for the exercise to be truly beneficial, you have to participate in it yourself. For kids who are overweight or who have already been diagnosed with diabetes, the psychological benefits of exercise may be of equal or greater importance than the physiological ones. The physiological benefits of exercise are immense as well, although certain precautions may be needed to prevent any diabetes-related problems from resulting from exercise.

The Physiological Benefits of Activity

Since it appears to be possible to control or essentially reverse diabetes with exercise alone, why aren't people convinced yet that exercise is essential? As with most things, maybe it is just that people need to be repeatedly hit over the head with a new idea before it finally sinks in. To prove the point yet again, another recent study, the Diabetes in Control 10,000 Step Study recruited people with type 2 diabetes and asked them to increase their physical activity *without* changing their diets. Participants had to be willing and committed to taking at least 10,000 steps throughout each day (equal to roughly five miles of walking), monitored with pedometers. A total of forty-four diabetic adults completed the study, clocking in over three million steps, the equivalent of almost 15,000 collective miles over three months. The conclusion: Diabetic adults wearing pedometers and with a daily goal to become more active all day (increasing from 3,100 steps up to 10,000) improved their physical fitness levels, blood sugars, cholesterol levels, blood pressure, and body weight; moreover, many of these improvements occurred after just the first four weeks of the study. By the end, over fifteen participants had reduced dosages of their various medications (including diabetes-related ones), six had completely eliminated some, and three had gone off all medications completely, despite a minimal average weight loss of only four pounds. So, I say again, if not a "cure" for diabetes, then exercise is surely the next best thing.

Whether prevention or an essential "reversal" of diabetes is possible in type 2 diabetic youth is a topic that remains largely unstudied. In adults with type 2 diabetes, we now know that regular exercise will likely decrease their insulin resistance and enable them to reduce or sometimes discontinue their diabetes medications. In kids, we know that excess body fat alone does not cause diabetes, but rather that an insurmountable insulin resistant state results mainly from their intake of refined sugars, high-GI foods, and unhealthy fat combined with their sedentary state and genetic risk. However, an unhealthy diet would assuredly not have the same negative impact on insulin action in a regularly active child whose exercise increases his or her insulin sensitivity; the relative glycemic effect of foods would be lower because this child's insulin would function more effectively to lower any glycemic spikes. In other words, an overweight but fit kid would better utilize carbohydrate just by having more insulin-responsive muscles. Thus, lack of exercise is also a potentially more potent contributor to diabetes development in our kids than misguided dietary choices.

Having said that, though, I must also point out that it makes sense that regular exercise done without any attention to eating right will have less of an influence on the prevention or control of diabetes than a combination of the two. For that reason, a quality diet is also an important component in treating our diabetic youth, and the two are best considered in concert—that is, daily activity *plus* a healthier diet.

As discussed, physical activity can have a huge effect on the action of insulin, and ineffective insulin is a universal problem in diabetic youth. Here's another way that exercise is beneficial to them in this regard: The only time their bodies can effectively handle high-GI and -GL foods is when they exercise long and/or hard. In those cases, a significant amount of the muscle glycogen is used up and intake of carbohydrates with a higher GI during the activity may actually be useful in providing their bodies with glucose to delay fatigue, particularly when exercising more than an hour. Following exercise, such carbohydrates can also be taken up from the bloodstream more easily for a couple of hours—with very little insulin needed—to replenish glycogen stores. During exercise, eating carbohydrate foods high in fat (like doughnuts) would not be appropriate, though, since fat slows the absorption of needed carbohydrates.

Carrying around extra body fat can pose a formidable challenge to being physically active, however. In fact, excessive weight can often keep kids from wanting to or being able to participate in sports or other physical pursuits. Being overweight, thus, potentially creates a "catch-22" for weight management because your children's nonparticipation in exercise due to their body size consequently lowers their daily calorie expenditure, which causes them to gain more fat weight. Don't give up on your kids being active, though. The next chapter will give you some helpful pointers for getting the most sedentary kids moving more.

While studies on type 2 diabetic kids and exercise are sparse, being physically active is still arguably the best "medicine" for youth with diabetes. In youth, whose pancreatic beta cell dysfunction has not been present as long, any improvement in insulin action in their bodies will lessen the stress on the pancreas to provide enough insulin as less of the hormone will be needed; couple that lower resistance due to activity with even minor dietary changes, and glycemic control may be readily achieved in youth.

Furthermore, exercise can likely prevent many of the complications related to poor glycemic control that people with diabetes face. Many of the diabetes-related complications (loss of sensation in the feet, eye disease, kidney problems, or heart disease) are related to having diabetes longer; thus, your child is at low risk for experiencing them simply due to his or her younger age. Nevertheless, diabetes by itself is an extremely strong risk factor for heart disease, and physical inactivity is also associated with a higher risk of dying from heart problems. With regular exercise, your child can improve blood sugars and virtually eliminate both heart disease risks at once.

Regular aerobic exercise also lessens the potential impact of most of the other cardiovascular risk factors, including elevated blood lipids (cholesterol and other blood fats), insulin resistance, obesity, and hypertension. High blood pressure is associated with higher levels of insulin, and regular physical activity can result in lower blood pressure *and* reduced circulating levels of insulin. If your child has elevated blood pressure, though, it is best for him or her to avoid certain higher-intensity or resistance exercises, which may cause blood pressure to rise dangerously high. Such activities include heavy weight training; near-maximal exercise of any type; activities that require intense, sustained contractions of the upper body like water skiing or windsurfing; or exercises that cause breath holding.

Even regular walking can keep your family from dying sooner, according to a recent study: Diabetic adults of all ages who walk at least two hours per week have a 39 percent lower risk of dying from any cause and a 34 percent reduction in their risk of dying from heart disease. People with diabetes also have a higher risk of joint-related injuries, so adoption of a moderate program of walking may be more suitable for most of them than a more vigorous exercise like running. That study also concluded that regular walking is likely the best medicine for both the prevention and treatment of type 2 diabetes.

Some of my own research on older people with type 2 diabetes has shown that the skin circulation in their feet—where they are at risk for developing ulcers—is slightly improved right after exercise and from regular aerobic exercise training. Good blood sugar control, when achieved with the help of regular physical activity, has the potential to prevent or delay almost all of the potential long-term health complications of diabetes.

One final concern is the prevention of dehydration during exercise. As elevated sugars can increase urinary water losses, your child's risk for losing excessive fluids is greater if blood sugars are not well controlled. Exercising itself compounds the risk by increasing sweating (thus loss of water), which can rapidly lead to a dehydrated state. Since exercising in the heat can be especially dangerous for kids—prepubescent ones in particular have a lesser ability to release heat through sweating—

adequate fluid replacement and frequent rest need to be high priorities. Have your child drink plenty of cool, plain water during and following such activities and take frequent breaks to have a chance to cool down, preferably out of the heat.

The Psychological Benefits of Being Active

Any individual with a chronic health problem can develop what I call a "chronic disease personality." Some people take on their health condition as a personal challenge, rising to do whatever is necessary or feasible to control it to the fullest extent possible. While such a proactive stance is generally helpful from a control standpoint, it can also lead people to become somewhat obsessive about their health and their daily care regimens, which may not be psychologically healthy. Others, however, respond in the opposite manner, acting as though their disease is nonexistent, which often leads them to ignore their health-care plan, forgo taking their prescribed medications, and disregard dietary and other recommendations that would improve their health status.

Regardless of the way your child has responded to his or her diagnosis of type 2 diabetes, he or she may have special emotional concerns that often arise in anyone dealing with an "incurable" chronic health condition. While diabetes may essentially be invisible to others, being overweight (like most kids with type 2 diabetes are) is clearly visible; either state, though—whether visible to peers or not—can wreak havoc on your child's emotional health and general psyche. No child feels good about being treated as physically inferior or even being shunned by peers, teachers, or coaches during PE, team sports, and other physical pursuits. Being the last one picked to play on a team can easily play into and worsen an overweight youth's already low self-esteem.

Here's how exercise comes in as the best "medicine" again. Many researchers have studied the psychological benefits of physical activity in people with and without chronic health conditions. The general consensus is that for everyone, regular exercise can relieve mild to moderate symptoms of depression and anxiety, as well as improve mood and self-perceptions. Particularly for girls, dissatisfaction with their bodies is associated with a lower self-esteem, and youth who perceive themselves as fat and out-of-shape are particularly vulnerable to a negative self-image. Kids today are even more susceptible to such bodily misperceptions because of television: Overweight teens who spend more time watching soap operas, movies, music videos, and sports reportedly have an even greater bodily dissatisfaction and drive for thinness. Exercise thus acts as "medicine" because it can improve body shape and size and, therefore, raise self-esteem and improve bodily satisfaction, particularly in overweight, diabetic youth.

The psychological benefits of regular aerobic exercise for adults have been well studied, but far less research has been conducted in youth. However, a recent study on teens' participation in endurance sports and their self-image found that regular endurance exercise was related to a more favorable self-image, as well as to improved psychological and physical well-being. By promoting physical fitness, lessening body mass, and resulting in a more favorable body shape, exercise leads to a greater acceptance by peers and an improved self-image in adolescents without diabetes. Kids with diabetes, therefore, have even more to gain psychologically with regular exercise.

Managing Blood Sugars Effectively During Exercise

Diabetic youth need to be well informed about the overall effect that exercise may have on their blood sugar control. Fortunately, with regular participation in any type of aerobic training, your child's enhanced insulin sensitivity alone will invariably improve his or her blood sugar control. While aerobic exercise generally has a moderate glucose-lowering effect, the acute response can vary. Moreover, depending on your child's medications (if any are taken), hypoglycemia (low blood sugar) can also potentially occur, as well as other diabetes-related problems and complications.

Managing blood sugars effectively with exercise requires a greater understanding of its effects on metabolism. As discussed, the type of exercise (easy, moderate, or intense) in which a diabetic youth engages has a big effect on glycemic responses, and intense activities can temporarily raise blood glucose levels. By using a mixture of fat, muscle glycogen, and blood glucose, prolonged activities seldom have that effect. Although mild activities like walking generally allow for more fat use, blood glucose use can become quite significant as muscle glycogen stores become depleted, increasing your child's risk (albeit small) of developing low blood sugar. Moreover, during higher-intensity, prolonged aerobic activities such as running (done at a greater than 65 percent of maximal capacity), carbohydrates are the body's exclusive fuel, and depletion of both muscle glycogen and blood glucose is inevitable if the activity lasts two or more hours. An intense activity such as repeated interval training results in significant depletion of muscle glycogen as well, thereby increasing blood glucose use and the risk of hypoglycemia for hours afterward.

Prolonged exercise in particular has a greater potential to cause hypoglycemia. If your child's diabetes is being controlled with diet and exercise alone, his or her risk of developing low blood sugar during exercise is minimal. Having your child consume a moderate amount (15 grams) of carbohydrate during and within thirty minutes after exhaustive, glycogen-depleting exercise lowers the risk of developing low blood sugar and allows for more efficient restoration of muscle glycogen after exercise. The risk is greater, though, if your child takes oral medications that lower blood glucose levels (primarily those that increase the pancreas's secretion of insulin, such as Amaryl or Glucotrol—please refer to medications in chapter 6), or if he or she is taking insulin injections.

Insulin use creates its own set of exercise concerns. If insulin is being used, extra care must be taken to prevent hypoglycemia because of the combined effects of exercise and insulin on glucose removal from the bloodstream. At rest, insulin alone facilitates the uptake of blood glucose into muscle and fat cells; during exercise, however, insulin levels decrease, and muscle contractions elicit glucose uptake directly—without insulin. Since the absorption and release of injected insulin cannot be "shut off" like your child's pancreas does with its own supply of insulin, more glucose will be taken up into the cells because of the additive uptake of glucose by muscle contractions *and* by this extra insulin. As a result, insulin users have a much greater risk of developing low blood sugar with exercise. To prevent this occurrence, diabetic exercisers need to check their blood sugar levels before, possibly during, and after exercise to monitor its effects and compensate by eating carbohydrate if blood sugars begin to drop too low.

For shorter duration and more intense activities, supplementing with a small amount of extra carbohydrates (5 to 10 grams) can effectively prevent blood sugars from dropping too much, but for your child to participate in more prolonged exercise training, you may need to consult with his or her diabetes health-care provider about reducing doses of oral medications or insulin (if either is taken) to prevent hypoglycemia. Alternately, for regular, planned exercise, you may be able to gauge how to effectively lower your child's pre-exercise insulin doses on your own (once the glycemic effects of the activity are determined) using a detailed, activity-specific guide for insulin users available in my first book, *The Diabetic Athlete*.

Your child can avoid developing severe hypoglycemia during physical activity with early recognition of its symptoms and rapid treatment. Hypoglycemia, usually defined as a blood glucose level less than 65 mg/dl (3.6 mM), requires immediate treatment when symptoms begin to occur; therefore, it is important to recognize its symptoms, listed in the table on page 112. Treat your child's low blood sugar immediately with small amounts (5 to 10 grams) of readily absorbed carbohydrates, such as you would find in two to three glucose tablets or pieces of hard candy, 3 to 4 ounces of regular soda or juice (the only good use for regular soda!), a handful of raisins, or a small serving of any high-GI food. Recheck blood sugars after five to ten minutes and consume more only if symptoms have not begun to resolve. Do not overtreat a low, or high blood sugar will be the rebound effect. Also, never treat hypoglycemia with chocolate, doughnuts, other high-fat sugary foods, or slowly absorbed, low-GI carbohydrates (such as whole-grain breads and most whole fruits) as they do not act rapidly enough for effective treatment.

So, without the additional caloric expenditure and other physical benefits that regular exercise provides, dieters are doomed to regain their lost weight (and more), and the rest of us can look forward to fat weight gain in the future. The time to start preventing and reversing these occurrences is now. Kids who participate in organized youth sports are significantly more likely to be physically active adults.

Common Symptoms of Hypoglycemia

•

- Cold or clammy skin
- Dizziness or lightheadedness
- Double or blurred vision
- Elevated pulse rate
- Headache
- Inability to do basic math
- Insomnia
- Irritability
- Mental confusion
- Nausea

- Nightmares
- Poor physical coordination
- Rapid-onset fatigue
- Shakiness
- Shaky hands
- Sweating
- Tingling of hands or tongue
- Tiredness
- Visual spots
- Weakness

Any physical activity, no matter how minor, is better than none for improving insulin action, lowering body fat, and increasing amounts of metabolically active muscle. Undeniably, when regular exercise is begun in the early stages of type 2 diabetes, your child can essentially make the condition disappear. So, what are you waiting for? Rush on to read the next chapter to learn how to incorporate more exercise into your kids' daily lives.

DAILY PHYSICAL ACTIVITIES

O
UR CURRENT societal struggle to increase our nation's level of physical activity reminds me of a bumper sticker I once saw that proudly proclaimed, "I'm in no shape to exercise!" If I had to create one to display on my bumper, mine would probably say, "Couch potatoes, arise and exercise!" Believe it or not, until your family starts exercising, you may not discover how bad being physically inactive actually makes you feel. Your family's frequent complaints of "being too tired to exercise" will virtually disappear once you become regularly physically active, and your energy levels will soar while your insulin resistance drops.

People often ask me how I manage to handle a full-time professorial job, research grants, book writing, lecturing, marriage, and a family (three active boys), and my response invariably is, "I work out." By exercising regularly, I keep myself from experiencing the sluggishness that generally accompanies an insulin resistant state, which everyone will develop from a sedentary lifestyle, and at the same time, I increase my endurance capacity so that I can go through each day with more energy to accomplish everything I need to.

We all know that most adults could use more exercise, but why are today's youth so inactive as well? Aren't kids supposed to be the ones who run ahead and wait for us tired older folks to catch up? This chapter will discuss the phenomenon of inactivity in youth before giving you numerous tips and activities to get your own youngsters moving more as painlessly (for you) as possible—starting today!

Inactivity of Youth Today

The honest, but disturbing, answer to how much exercise kids are actually getting nowadays is, "Not nearly enough!" Have you ever found yourself saying to your kids, "Don't just sit there—get up and do something!" or "Go outside and get some exercise!" just to get them away from the TV? According to the latest statistics, saying that is akin to telling them, "Do what I say, not what I do," for the majority of us, which seldom works. The new millennium began with more than 60 percent of all American adults (parents included) not being regularly physically active, and a quarter of them not exercising at all in spite of its widely broadcast health benefits.

Causes of Physical Inactivity

Obviously, knowing that exercise is good for you is not enough to motivate everyone to do it, and as far as your kids go, assume that they are much more likely to follow your lead than what you preach (especially if you are not a physically active role model yourself). Is it any wonder then that, on the whole, our kids are inactive as well? Adults may unconsciously be even more of the problem than being a poor role model. For instance, ask yourself how many times you unthinkingly strapped your infant, toddler, or preschooler into his or her stroller, effectively trapping your child into a sedentary state for your own convenience or to save time? Such physical restraint of children by adults generally continues as they grow older as well, manifesting whenever you attempt to control their behavior by making them sit quietly for long periods of time, be it in school, in the car, or in your home.

In fact, a recent study assessing the eating and exercise habits of al-

U.S. Surgeon General's Report (2000)

•

According to the latest U.S. Surgeon General's report, here's how truly widespread the problem of physical inactivity has become among our children:

- Nearly 50 percent of America's youth between the ages of twelve and twenty-one never participate in *any* vigorous physical activity
- About 14 percent of our youth do not exercise at all, with inactivity predominating in females (14 percent) compared to males (7 percent), as well as in African American females (21 percent) compared to Caucasian ones (12 percent)
- Participation in any type of physical activity among our youth lessens dramatically with advancing age or grade in school
- Less than 20 percent of all high school students are physically active enough to meet the minimum recommendation of twenty minutes of activity, five days a week, in physical education classes
- In the early 1990s, daily participation in physical education classes dropped by 17 percent (from 42 percent down to 25 percent four years later)

most 900 children concluded that lack of physical activity—particularly vigorous exercise—is likely the most significant contributor to childhood obesity. Combined with too much time being spent on sedentary behaviors like computer games and TV watching, insufficient exercise may equal or exceed diet quality as a contributor to weight gain, particularly among teens.

The removal of consistent physical education classes from many school curricula in order to focus on better student performance on government-mandated standards of learning (SOL) in academic subjects is occurring at the worst possible time—when inexpensive and nutritionally poor consumables are available to our youth in ever-increasing portions. Many schools now offer very limited PE classes (once or twice a week rather than daily in elementary schools), or even none at all. The only glimmer of hope in this situation is that some schools are beginning to implement the "new" PE, characterized by participation in a wide variety of physical activities (including rock climbing) rather than competition. In times past, overweight children have been shunned during competitive play and made to feel even more self-conscious about their excess body weight, which only contributes to the problem.

Nevertheless, our kids' overall level of inactivity has escalated even more dramatically now that they are not only less active in school, but are also replacing their physically active leisure-time pursuits with sedentary ones like surfing the Net, playing computer and other video games, and watching countless hours of television (with literally hundreds of channels to peruse). Fewer kids, on the whole, are participating in after-school sports and other physically active extracurricular pursuits.

Although a lot of sitting around for any reason is best avoided, TV watching appears to be especially detrimental because your rate of energy expenditure (metabolic rate) is even lower during this sedentary pursuit than during other sit-down activities, such as playing board games or even reading. Many pediatricians are now recommending that children be restricted from spending more than one to two hours a day using TVs and computers combined (although extra time on the computer may be allowed as needed for homework). Kids who watch a lot of TV are also more likely to have bad eating habits, such as munching on unhealthy, high-calorie snacks while watching, likely driven by the many junk food commercials targeting youth. In fact, a longitudinal study recently revealed that the amount of TV watched during childhood and adolescence is directly associated with the risk of high cholesterol, diabetes, poor fitness, smoking, and obesity in adulthood.

Physical Activities for Youth

To choose the right exercise for kids, start by forgetting the "no pain, no gain" mentality perpetually circulating around fitness clubs and gyms; in fact, an uncomfortable amount of discomfort in exercising muscles is not even necessary for adults to achieve substantial gains in health or fitness. Physical adaptations to exercise can occur with very moderate intensity exercise, and even more importantly, every type of physical activity expends some calories.

The Surgeon General recently recommended moderate amounts of daily physical activity for people of all ages comprised of thirty minutes of moderate activities (like brisk walking) or shorter sessions of more intense exercise, including jogging or playing basketball for fifteen to twenty minutes. Of course, engaging in even more total physical activity may offer additional benefits, but only up to a point. Excessive exercise (such as ninety minutes or more daily of moderate- or high-intensity exercise) should be avoided by kids in particular to prevent potential injuries to maturing bones, joints, and muscles. Even in adults, the incidence of so-called "overuse injuries," such as inflamed tendons (tendinitis) and stress fractures in bones, soars when more than sixty to ninety minutes of hard exercise is done daily.

Physical Immaturity of Youth

You should never consider your children to be miniature adults. It is not just their smaller size that makes them dissimilar; physiologically speaking, they are quite unlike us more mature folks. Exercise programs for our youth, therefore, should be designed to meet the unique physiology of their growing, maturing bodies. When reenacting the proverbial "tortoise and the hare" scenario while walking with your kids—the one where you plod along at one continuous pace like the tortoise while your child sprints ahead like a jackrabbit, but then frequently stops and waits for you to catch up—your family is, in essence, simply doing what you all are best adapted to do, based on your physiology. To be safe and effective, their exercise participation needs to be designed to accommodate these distinctions.

Until children go through their final growth spurt and reach puberty, their bodies are not fully mature. Their bones are not fully calcified; their nervous systems and muscles are immature; their ability to generate energy (ATP) from muscle glycogen stores is limited; and their ability to thermoregulate, or adequately heat and cool themselves, is somewhat limited.

For starters, the immaturity of their bones, nerves, and muscles makes it impossible for resistance (weight) training to cause significant gains in strength before late adolescence (when they have gone through puberty). Moreover, heavy weight training in prepubescent youngsters has the capacity to injure the growth plates in the long bones, which could stunt their longitudinal growth. Overuse of certain joints by children such as the shoulder caused by repeated excessive throwing motions (as in softball or baseball) can damage the rotator cuff muscles and surrounding joint structures and should be avoided (this is why the number of pitches that Little Leaguers are now allowed to throw is limited). In addition, prepubescent youth should not engage in excessive amounts of endurance training as it may negatively affect bone maturation and health by causing loss of calcium from bones at a time when they should be depositing more.

Next, the immaturity of children's energy systems explains their stop-and-start version of physical activity. Kids can effectively use the first energy system, which is comprised of phosphagens like ATP and creatine phosphate stored in muscle (hence their propensity to sprint ahead), but activities that are slightly longer are much harder for them to do as their lactic acid energy system (used for exercise lasting thirty seconds to two minutes) is limited by smaller muscle glycogen stores, making this system somewhat ineffective until they reach puberty. As for endurance exercise, prepubescent youngsters use relatively more blood sugar and less stored glycogen during moderate exercise, so taking in carbohydrate drinks during extended activities (such as running, soccer, and swimming) may be necessary for kids to continue to participate at full tilt; however, kids may be better adapted for fat use than adults and appear to be well suited for prolonged exercise—as long as it is moderate or lower intensity in nature.

Finally, since immature sweat glands limit children's ability to sweat to cool down, special precautions must be taken to prevent them from overheating during activities, especially when done on warmer days. It is very important to give them adequate amounts of cool fluids during exercise and more frequent periods of rest (preferably out of the sun) than an adult would need during similar activities. Also, have them wear white or light-colored clothing to deflect some of the radiant heat from the sun. Conversely, kids can also chill more easily than adults during outdoor activities in the cold—sitting on the bench or sidelined for some reason during sporting events—especially if a child is inactive.

Suggested Daily Physical Activities

A physical activity pyramid (similar in concept to the food guide) has been created to give general recommendations for appropriate daily

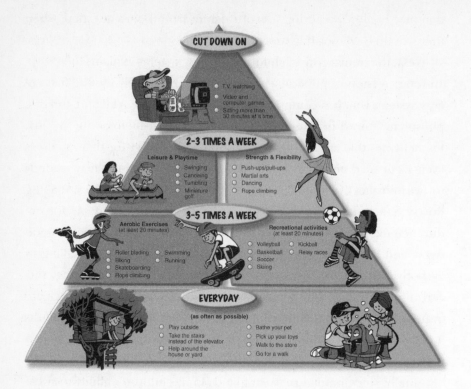

Copyright © 2003 by University of Missouri.
Published by MU Extension, University of Missouri-Columbia.

physical activity for adults, and may also be appropriate for teens who have gone through puberty. Given prepubescent children's physiological differences and typical leisure-type activities, though, modifications from the adult pyramid are needed for school-age children. One such pyramid has been created and is pictured in the figure above.

As you can see, the base of this modified pyramid recommends that children be as active as possible on a daily basis doing activities such as playing outside, walking, and helping around the house. These activities are the equivalent of "unstructured" physical activities, or ones that they are engaging in just in the course of being kids. The next higher level recommends twenty minutes of aerobic exercise or recreational sports three to five days per week, which includes more "structured" (planned) activities such as biking, Rollerblading, kickball, and organized sports. Listed in the two to three days per week range are strength and flexibility activities such as pull-ups, push-ups, martial arts, and rope climbing, as well as low-level leisure activities like swinging or miniature golf. Finally, it recommends cutting down on all sedentary pursuits, including TV watching, computer and video games, and sitting for more than thirty minutes at a time for any reason.

Despite the fact that playing outdoors is recommended daily and should equate to being physically active, I personally have had problems with getting my own kids to always approach it that way. In particular, I remember one time when I instructed my then six-year-old son to go outside and play, only to discover him twenty minutes later sitting on the curb next to a neighbor boy and watching the other boy play with his GameBoy. I never expected that outcome from my request that he go "play outdoors," but it certainly exemplifies the fact that it is important to practice what you preach by getting the whole family involved in being physically active. What I should have done instead of sending him outside to play by himself was take the time to go outdoors with my son, either to play catch, kick around a soccer ball in the yard, go for a bike ride, or take a walk around the neighborhood together.

Speaking of being active as a family, walking—either as a structured exercise, or just increasing the number of steps that you take during the day—is an activity from which every member of your family can benefit. It is the most popular leisure-time physical activity among adults, followed by gardening and yard work (the latter two would definitely not rank on most kids' list of fun activities, though). Generally, walking expends about one calorie per kilogram (kg) of body weight (pounds divided by 2.2 equals kg) per kilometer (about 0.6 miles) when you walk at a speed of two to four miles per hour, or for a 60 kg (130 lb) person, about 100 calories are used up per mile. Only 2,000 steps a day equals about a mile, which for most overweight adults and teens expends well more than 100 extra calories because of their heavier bodies.

Previously, researchers believed that exercise had to be vigorous to bestow meaningful health benefits, but more recently, a study conducted at Harvard found that, for adult women at least, moderate (brisk) walking decreased their risk for developing diabetes to the same degree as participation in vigorous activity. Simply being physically active during their leisure time—particularly if doing longer or more intense activities—by itself also reduced their diabetes risk as well. In other words, as far as your health is concerned, what really matters is expending those extra calories any way that you can.

Adding extra steps throughout the day will be well worth the effort. To get your family started walking more, simply try to emphasize it in an unstructured way that fits into your family's busy schedule. Additional walking can be added into your family's daily routine more easily than you can imagine. For example, try taking a flight of steps with your kids instead of the elevator or an escalator whenever possible, or at least walk up or down the escalator instead of standing while it does the work for you. If going up steps is too hard, then start with only walking down. Another good idea is to hide the remote to your TV so that your kids have to get up to change the channel. Also, make it a family rule that everyone has to walk around for five minutes after every thirty minutes of a sedentary activity.

If motivation is your family's biggest problem, do fun things like making a game out of trying to count how many steps you take a day. Based on the 10,000 Steps Study mentioned previously, it appears that we could all benefit immensely from taking at least that many steps throughout each day. If nothing else, helping your kids become more conscious of how active they are (or are not) during the day may assist them in remembering to add in more steps whenever possible. You may want to consider going out and investing in an inexpensive pedometer for them to use as additional motivation. Believe me, most kids will actually think they are fun to use (mine do)!

Maybe walking is not your kids' cup of tea, and they would rather take a family bike ride. That's okay, too, but keep in mind that cycling expends

Finding Motivation in Counting Your Daily Steps

•

A national campaign called America on the Move is currently advocating the same increase in steps (2,000 more per day) to be taken by everyone. For more information on this campaign and to use their free online step tracker, access their Web site at www.americaonthemove.org.

In addition, the American Diabetes Association sponsors Club Ped, an online group that your family can join to keep track of your steps, your progress, and your step goals. All you will need to get started is a pedometer (step counter). Club Ped can be accessed at www.diabetes .org/ClubPed/index.jsp.

Numerous other pedometer-based walking programs are available and can be accessed online at Web sites such as the following:

• AccuSplit pedometer company: www.accustep10000.org
• Step Tracker.com: www.steptracker.com
• About Walking.com: www.walking.about.com

Inexpensive pedometers can be purchased through sporting good stores or ordered online from various Web sites, including www.americaon themove.org, www.accusplit.com, www.digiwalker.com, www.walk4life.com, and www.pedometersusa.com. New-Lifestyles.com (www.new-lifestyles .com) also offers school pedometer kits that come in packs of fifteen or thirty through its link at www.thepedometercompany.com/digischool .html.

only a third of the energy you use walking the same distance, so your family would have to bike about three miles to equal the energy spent walking just one. Doing either activity, though, your kids are expending calories.

Unlike some adults, children seldom exert themselves solely for the health benefits of exercise; rather, they usually need some other gratification from participating, such as enjoyment. (Actually, most adults need exercise to be fun, too, or they would not continue to do it over the long haul.) If exercising becomes an integrated part of your lifestyle, it is more likely to be maintained long term. For motivation, try using a sticker chart to keep a visible account of physical activities that are accomplished each day by everyone in the family, and use frequent reinforcement with "tokens" or "treats" when goals are met. Such rewards, though, should seldom be comprised of caloric treats. Instead, try an outing to somewhere special, the purchase of a coveted toy or item, or anything else that is reasonable and effectively motivates your kids.

Helpful recommendations for physical activities, activity logs, and other motivational tools are widely available (but underutilized). For youth, some good sources of such tools are The President's Council on Physical Fitness and Sports (www.fitness.gov), The President's Challenge— Physical Activity and Fitness Awards Program (www.presidentschallenge .org), and Canada's Physical Activity Guides for Children and Youth (www.hc-sc.gc.ca/hppb/paguide/child_youth/index.html). Ten helpful ideas for kids and adults to get active from the President's Challenge follow on page 127.

Unstructured vs. Structured Activities

Getting your family motivated to be more physically active may not be nearly as hard as you may think. It really just requires that you start to think more broadly about what constitutes exercise, as you can see from the following ideas to get active. Stop trying to find the closest parking spot, using the remote control, and waiting for the elevator when you could be using the stairs. Simply adding a dozen steps here and there can easily add up to a substantial number over the course of the day and suffice to prevent insulin resistance and weight gain. Other helpful suggestions about how to increase both structured and unstructured physical activity on a daily basis, including recommended activities for your kids, are also given on the following pages.

Ideas for Younger Kids to Get Active

•

- Take your dog out for a walk
- Start up a playground kickball game
- Join a sports team
- Go to the park with a friend
- Help your parents with yard work
- Play tag with kids in your neighborhood
- Ride your bike to school
- Walk to the store for your mom
- See how many jumping jacks you can do
- Race a friend to the end of the block

Ideas for Adults (and Older Teens)

•

- Use a push mower to mow the lawn
- Go for a walk in a nearby park
- Take the stairs instead of an elevator
- Bike to work, to run errands, or to visit friends
- Clean out the garage or the attic
- Walk with a friend over the lunch hour
- Volunteer to become a coach or referee
- Sign up for a group exercise class
- Join a softball league
- Park at the farthest end of the lot

The President's Challenge (www.presidentschallenge.org/tools_ to_help/ten_ideas.aspx).

Tips for Adding Unstructured Exercise

•

- Add as many additional steps as possible (minimally 2,000) every day by having your children walk whenever and wherever they can
- Whenever your kids have ten free minutes, encourage them to walk around instead of sitting down
- Always take the stairs instead of the elevator or escalator
- Get your kids more involved in helping doing physical chores around the house, like cleaning, sweeping, mopping, vacuuming, and washing dishes
- Make a game out of raking the leaves in the yard
- Take your kids with you when shopping for groceries (as an added bonus, use the time to teach them about which foods are healthier to eat)
- Take your kids window shopping at the nearest mall
- Blow up a balloon and hit it around the house with your kids
- Put on some music and have an impromptu family dance
- Send your kids outside to kick or hit a ball around or throw a Frisbee
- Get a basketball hoop to set up in your driveway and send your kids outside to play regularly, or walk to the nearest neighborhood school and use theirs
- On nice days, take your kids to the nearest park to walk or play
- Encourage your kids to take the dog out for a daily walk (dogs need exercise, too!)
- Remember to have the whole family get up and move around after every thirty minutes of sedentary activity
- Always have your kids walk around while talking on the telephone
- Hide the remote for the TV, stereo, and other devices
- Have your kids walk in place, dance, or simply move while watching TV—at least during the commercial breaks
- Alternatively, invest in a rebounder (mini-trampoline) and have them jump while watching
- Limit your kids' TV and computer use to no more than two hours per day, or at least reduce their use by a minimum of thirty minutes daily

As for structured exercise like participation on sports teams or workouts using exercise equipment, many people find this type of activity harder to consistently fit into their daily routines. Most kids at least occasionally have after-school activities (not necessarily physically active ones, though), evening meetings, excessive amounts of homework, social activities, or other time-consuming events that may limit their ability to consistently exercise in a "structured" way during their leisure time. Your kids are not alone, though: Studies have shown that people

Tips for Adding Structured Exercise

•

- For teenagers, try to have them add at least thirty minutes of any type of physical activity to each day
- Encourage your children to sign up for an after-school team activity like soccer, baseball, basketball, or gymnastics
- During the off-season from a usual school sport, have them participate in another one, or find a league not affiliated with their school that practices, then
- Get the whole family involved in community physical activities, such as fun runs and walks
- Find the nearest tennis court and encourage your kids to start playing regularly (have them take lessons, if needed)
- Have your kids register for PE classes at school, even in high school
- Go for family walks whenever possible on weekends or in the evenings
- Set aside fifteen to twenty minutes a day after homework is done to walk, run, or jump in place as a family while your kids talk about their day
- Instead of driving, have your children walk, run, or bike wherever they need to go whenever possible
- Teach your kids how to safely use your (dusty!) home exercise equipment, particularly stationary bikes, treadmills, rebounders, or rowers

are more likely to consistently accumulate the recommended amounts of physical activity during the day by increasing their unstructured activities than with a formal exercise program due primarily to time constraints. Also, a higher level of motivation is needed to continue participating in structured exercise over time, and rates of continued participation are notoriously abysmal. Still, structured exercise undeniably has its benefits and remains highly recommended for overall good health and a higher level of physical fitness. If your family cannot manage to do regular workouts consistently, though, then it pays as a minimum to emphasize the unstructured ones on a daily basis.

Another practice to enhance overall fitness and insulin sensitivity is to incorporate workouts of varying intensities into your family's weekly routine. For example, it is better for a number of physiological (as well as psychological) reasons to alternate easy and hard workouts, especially once teens have finished their final growing spurt during puberty. Almost all seasoned athletes vary their training in this manner and for good reason. In order for anyone's body to fully recover from intense workouts, it needs adequate rest, which includes not just proper amounts of sleep, but also enough time between workouts to fully rebuild and recuperate. Easy workouts do not cause the same level of glycogen depletion and muscle damage as harder ones and thus constitute a form of "rest" by themselves. By alternating workout intensities, your kids' bodies get both the enhanced fitness benefits attributable to hard workouts and the healing effects of greater recuperative time between intense workouts. Doing so also helps prevent "overuse syndrome," which includes more frequent colds, chronic tiredness, and joint and muscle injuries.

Additional Strategies for Motivating Overweight Kids

Overweight and obese children have special concerns about structured exercise routines. In particular, these kids may be acutely aware of their larger body size, making them more self-conscious during such activities or preventing them from wanting to participate at all. If your child fits this profile, it is especially important for you to help him or her find activities that are perceived as enjoyable to have any hope of continued participation. Your child may need to try out a few different activities until favored ones can be found, but doing so will be well worth the extra effort.

Ideally, structured programs for overweight kids should involve activities that allow them to move their whole bodies over the greatest distance possible to maximize their energy expenditure. However, although walking and jogging fall into this category of activities, most kids will find them either boring or too difficult. You can trick your kids into walking more simply by incorporating it into other activities—like parking farther away than necessary when you take them shopping. Moreover, walking can be the gateway to more vigorous exercise for many overweight youth, which can further increase their overall health benefits. As a bonus, self-confidence may improve once they start a walking program, which may lead them to start including additional physical activities into their lives. Some more popular, but suitable, alternatives among the younger set include dancing, basketball, skating, and cycling.

Furthermore, the addition of supervised resistance (weight) training can bestow extra health benefits, especially in more mature teens. Such training increases muscle mass, which can enhance both their insulin action and their round-the-clock resting energy expenditure (and, thus, their glycemic control), not to mention their self-esteem and feelings of accomplishment. Measurable increases in strength can actually be attained in as short as one to two weeks (as neural changes occur before gains in muscle size), which may additionally motivate your child to continue moderate weight lifting. Boys, in particular, are more focused on gaining muscle, while girls are usually more interested in weight loss alone; however, girls also benefit from muscular gains, which may lead to greater fat weight loss despite potentially lower body weight losses.

It is further recommended that you build on your child's strong physical attributes. For example, most overweight children are on the top of the growth charts—usually both tall and strong. Consequently, they may be more likely to succeed in sports and activities involving height and strength, such as basketball, football, and field events like shot put and discus. However, they may also be lacking in speed and agility, which will limit their ability to excel in sports requiring these abilities, namely track, soccer, or jumping events.

Extra fat stored under the skin also acts to insulate them and keep them warmer in the pool, which is an advantage in pools heated to 80 degrees or less, as heat losses through the skin in water are usually much greater than they are in air. Also, the water serves to hide their bodies, which may decrease the inhibition that they may feel when their figures are more plainly seen during other activities.

Although we have touched on different ways to motivate your kids to be more physically active, you may still be at a loss as to how and where to start with your own kids. The most sedentary kids may be the most resistant to trying anything new. Just like when you make the transition to better eating, it will be easier for your family if you ease into being more active gradually. Walking more may be a great way to start, but moderation in all things is appropriate, which means that you need to start out slowly.

For example, you don't want to find yourself in a situation like one I witnessed recently in the Virginia mountains: My family had hiked straight down at least a mile-long footpath through the woods to reach some stunning waterfalls. Near the bottom, I passed a relatively lean parent trying to coax her visibly overweight, prepubescent teenage daughter back up the path and overheard the mother saying in an exasperated tone of voice, "What do you expect me to do? I can't just go get the car and drive down here to pick you up!" That family was literally and figuratively in for an uphill climb on the road to physical fitness.

So, what should you do? Plan big and start small. Try using the strategies already discussed to begin implementing more physical activity into your family's daily lives. If your kids boycott your attempts, then

Tips for Motivating the Most Sedentary Kids

•

- Start with a five-minute rule: Tell your kids they have to be physically active for five minutes; if they want to stop after five, let them (they may not)
- Insist that your kids routinely get up and move around during TV commercials; progress toward having them walk or even dance during that time
- Make your kids get up and move around for three to five minutes at the end of every thirty minutes of sedentary activity (even when reading or doing homework)
- Turn the TV and all electronic devices off for a specified period of time every day, thus limiting the time your kids spend in front of them
- Remove all TVs from your kids' bedrooms, as having them there promotes even greater physical inactivity
- Set time limits for all sedentary activities, and use planned physical activities (like bowling or roller skating) to reward your kids' accomplishments
- Buy your kids toys that promote physical activity (like skates or a bike) instead of toys that promote sitting and inactivity
- Steer your kids toward doing at least one physically active chore around the house or yard daily, like sweeping, vacuuming, or raking leaves
- Make up a daily physical activity chart that your youngsters can use to record their time spent being active, and set up a system of noncaloric rewards
- Do whatever you can to be an active role model; your kids may see you doing something that looks like fun and want to join in

try some of the additional tips given to smooth the transition toward greater physical activity.

Of course, it would be optimal for your kids to always be regular about their physical activity (doing more structured activities at least three days per week); realistically, though, we act as the role models and facilitators of an active lifestyle for our kids, and many of us are not good at that particular parental job. In lieu of imposing a potentially unsustainable exercise program on our kids, we would do better to simply model adding in physical activity at every opportunity.

Be willing to try just about anything as every little bit of extra movement that your kids do during every day counts. Just to illustrate how easy it really is for your kids to become more physically active, a sample plan for children appears on the following page.

For teenagers, a similar plan can be implemented with minor adjustments. For example, if talking on the phone with friends instead of watching TV, encourage your teens to walk around rather than sitting. Also, if shut up in their rooms with the music blaring, encourage them to dance along with it. Teens may also be more amenable to adding in some light resistance exercises using dumbbells or resistance bands to start; after feeling more comfortable with the weights, they may even agree to join a fitness club to use their weight machines and other fitness equipment. You may also want to dust off your exercise bike, rower, or treadmill and encourage your kids to exercise during their favorite TV shows or movies. If they sleep late on weekends, encourage them to add fifteen minutes of activity for each extra hour of sleep over eight or nine hours later in the day to compensate. (Energy use is lowest during sleep; even sitting while awake uses more calories.)

Keep in mind that any plan that I could suggest will undoubtedly have to be modified to meet your kids' preferences and your family's lifestyle. Listing every possible physical activity is beyond the scope of this book; however, books, articles, and videos giving ideas and techniques for stretching, easy calisthenics, resistance training, aerobic exercise, and other physical activities are abundant both in stores and on

Sample Increased Physical Activity Plan
(for Children Ages Five to Twelve)

•

Weekdays

Upon awakening Completely tense whole body and relax ten times (1 to 2 minutes)

Upon rising Do warm-up exercises ten times each (toe touches, side bends, trunk twists, arm circles, neck rolls, knee lifts, calf stretches, jumping jacks) (5 minutes)

On the way to school Either be dropped off a block away from school or arrive at the bus stop 5 minutes early and walk back and forth while waiting (5 minutes)

After school As soon as arrive home, walk around the house five extra times before entering; if weather is inclement, walk around inside (5 minutes)

While doing homework Walk around, jump, or dance for 5 minutes after every 15 to 20 minutes of homework (and/or go up and down stairs, if there are any) (5 to 15 minutes)

Before dinner Help set the table, fill up drink glasses, or fix dinner (5 minutes)

After dinner Help clear the table and do dishes (or load the dishwasher) (5 minutes)

During evening leisure time Walk in place or jump during every TV commercial; if using computer games, do the same for 5 minutes out of every half hour (10 to 20 minutes)

Before bedtime Raise and lower up on balls of your feet while brushing teeth; raise and lower elbows while flossing (4 to 5 minutes)

Weekdays: *Minimum* added physical activity is 45 minutes a day

Weekends

Upon awakening Completely tense whole body and relax ten times (1 to 2 minutes)

Upon rising Do warm-up exercises ten times each (toe touches, side bends, trunk twists, arm circles, neck rolls, knee lifts, calf stretches, jumping jacks) (5 minutes)

During morning cartoon time Walk in place or jump during every TV commercial; if using computer or video games, do the same for 5 minutes out of every half hour (20 to 30 minutes)

Before lunch Take the dog out for a walk with a parent (30 minutes)

After lunch Go (window) shopping with a parent, older sibling, or friend; park farther away on purpose, take the stairs, walk on escalators, etc. Alternately, go to the park for a family walk, bike ride, or other recreation (40 to 60+ minutes)

Before dinner Help vacuum, sweep, or clean up around the house (5 minutes)

After dinner Turn on the stereo and dance to your favorite song (5 minutes)

During evening leisure time Walk in place or jump during every TV commercial; if using computer games, do the same for 5 minutes out of every half hour (10 to 20 minutes)

Before bedtime Raise and lower up on balls of your feet while brushing teeth; raise and lower elbows while flossing (4 to 5 minutes)

Weekends: *Minimum* added physical activity is 120 minutes a day

the Internet. For additional ideas on how to make anything you or your kids do during the day more physically active, I also recommend consulting a book called *The Anytime, Anywhere Exercise Book.*

Finally, the list on pages 137–38 contains additional activities that can be implemented anytime to increase the physical activity of the most sedentary—and most resistant—kids. The joy of these activities is that they can often be undertaken without your kids even realizing that they are being more active.

So, it's finally time for your family to lose all its excuses, get up off the couch, and start being more physically active. As previously mentioned, an easy way is to simply start by trying to add 2,000 extra steps (about one mile) to every day in an unstructured way. As your kids begin to feel the positive effects of this extra movement on their fitness level, try out some structured activities until you can find one or more that both fits your kids' limited time and is enjoyable. If possible, make them family activities to give your reluctant teen the encouragement that he or she needs to continue being active. Whatever you and your kids do to increase your daily exercise, though—be it structured or unstructured—focus on making it a permanent, healthy addition to your daily lives.

Additional Activities for the Most Sedentary Kids

•

- Put an emphasis on playing and recreating, rather than exercising
- Show your kids some basic flexibility and warm-up exercises (toe touches, side bends, trunk twists, arm circles, neck rolls, knee lifts, calf stretches, etc.), and encourage them to take a few minutes every day to do at least some of them
- Put your child in charge of teaching the whole family a new physical activity that he or she learned at school or elsewhere
- Use some sidewalk chalk to play hopscotch with your kids
- Play hide-and-seek with your kids, indoors and outdoors
- Plant and tend a garden together with your kids; they may be more willing to eat vegetables that they help grow
- Have your kids throw a ball or Frisbee in the yard for a dog
- Teach your child how to fly a kite on a windy day

- Send the kids to summer camp (daily or overnight)
- When they are ready for part-time jobs, help your kids find ones to keep them active (lawn care, newspaper delivery, caddy, waiter or bus-boy, etc.)
- Whenever you need to have a serious talk with your teens (or younger kids), take them out for a walk to do it
- Involve your kids in a fund-raising walk for your favorite charity and collect donations based on the number of miles they walk
- Adopt an elderly neighbor or relative who could use your kids' help with some chores around the house and yard
- If school is not prohibitively far away, take the extra time to walk your kids to school instead of driving or busing them there

6

DIABETIC MEDICATIONS AND OTHER SUPPLEMENTS

WE HAVE ALREADY discussed the first two cornerstones of diabetes management—diet and exercise—at length, leaving only the third and final one: medications. Remember that "miracle pill" from the first chapter—the one you could give your child every day as a cure? The new instructions are simple: Take that pill every day, put it in your child's pocket, and ensure that he or she takes it for a walk, out for a bike ride, to the park to play, to after-school soccer practices, to the swimming pool, or to do anything physically active for at least thirty minutes a day. Do you realize that if every parent could accomplish that, chances are that there truly would be no more type 2 diabetes in kids? As we know all too well, though, such a feat is easier said than done. Since that scenario is not likely to happen for a lot of reasons, a discussion of what prescribed medications and other dietary supplements can do for your child's diabetes control and overall health is in order.

Third Cornerstone in Diabetes Management

Diabetic medications as the third cornerstone in diabetes management, along with changes in food intake and sedentary behaviors, can be vitally important in the battle to effectively control your child's blood sugar levels. Think of it this way: Medications are a way to potentially enhance the benefits that your child is gaining from other lifestyle changes, particularly if those changes are not controlling diabetes on their own. The three cornerstones should ideally be viewed as three separate but interrelated weapons in the battle to win the "war" against diabetes.

The American Diabetes Association's (ADA) position statement on type 2 diabetes in children and adolescents asserts that the ideal goal of treatment for kids is normalization of blood glucose levels, similar to adults with type 2. Glycemic control should be accomplished through self-management education for parent and child that includes learning how to use a blood glucose meter at home, meeting with a registered dietitian who works with kids with diabetes, possibly gathering more information through peer support groups and diabetes camps, being encouraged to participate in more daily physical activities, and using medications if blood sugar control is not achieved with the former strategies. Your child's diabetes health-care team should make the decisions about when medications are necessary and which ones to use.

Oral Medications

When does your child need to start taking diabetic medications? Ideally, they should only be initiated after the first two treatment modalities have been attempted and failed to satisfactorily control your child's blood glucose levels. The ADA defines successful treatment with diet and exercise in youth as "cessation of excessive weight gain with normal linear growth, near-normal fasting blood glucose values (less than 125 mg/dl), and near normal glycated hemoglobin (HbA_{1c}) levels." As previously mentioned, the latter is an excellent indicator of overall glucose control over the previous two to three months (particularly, the prior month) and is determined with a simple blood draw; a value of less than 6.5 to 7.0 percent (in most labs) would be the ultimate goal. If diabetes control is not adequate, then initiation of medications is the next step.

While not much research on successful treatment of diabetic kids is currently available, in adults the results are not encouraging: Over time, fewer than 10 percent of them are able to successfully manage their diabetes with lifestyle changes alone without resorting to oral diabetic medications or insulin. Type 2 diabetes appears to be progressive, with worsening glycemic control over time even with good adherence to dietary and lifestyle improvements; this outcome is likely the result of extensive failure of the insulin-producing beta cells of the pancreas. For kids diagnosed with the condition, though, the fact that they are young and have stressed their beta cells by overproducing insulin for significantly fewer years than the typical adult with diabetes may give type 2 diabetic youth a greater chance of achieving control with a combination of good dietary habits, regular physical activity, and glucose-lowering medications.

If your child has been prescribed an oral diabetic medication for his or her diabetes treatment, it comes from one of five classes of drugs currently approved to treat type 2 diabetes in the United States. Although none of these drugs is currently approved by the FDA for use in youth, they are assumed to be similarly effective and safe to use since the pathophysiology of diabetes in children and adolescents appears to be similar to adults. The five classes are detailed in the table that follows.

The first class of drugs recommended for diabetic youth is the biguanides, of which Glucophage is the only one with FDA approval for

Current Oral Diabetic Medications

Class of Drug	Examples (Brand Name)	Mechanism of Action(s)
Biguanides	Glucophage	↓ liver glucose output, ↑ liver and muscle insulin sensitivity, but no direct effect on beta cells
Sulfonylureas	Amaryl, DiaBeta, Glynase, Glucotrol, Glyburide, Micronase	Promote insulin secretion from the beta cells of the pancreas; some may ↑ insulin sensitivity
Meglitinides	Prandin, Starlix	Stimulates beta cells to increase insulin secretion (for a very short duration)
Thiazolidenediones	Avandia, Actos	↑ insulin sensitivity of peripheral tissues, such as muscle
Alpha-Glucosidase Inhibitors	Precose, Glyset	Works in intestines to slow conversion of ingested carbohydrates to simple sugars

use (in adults). Adult doses are normally prescribed for youth because most diabetic teens are near or at adult body weights. Its primary advantage over sulfonylureas (e.g., DiaBeta and Glucotrol) is that it cannot induce hypoglycemia (low blood sugar); rather, it exerts its effects by shutting down the liver's excessive production of glucose overnight and by improving insulin action in both liver and muscle tissues. It is also the only diabetes medication that promotes weight loss, which is another good reason to use it as a first-line drug. Finally, Glucophage appears to be somewhat heart protective as people taking it have also been found to survive longer than others taking alternate diabetic medications.

Glucophage is not without potential side effects, though. Mild nausea and diarrhea are common among its users, but taking it with meals generally decreases these symptoms. Many people are more tolerant of the sustained release preparation of this medication (Glucophage XR). During acute illness, its use may have to be discontinued, however, as it may induce a state of lactic acidosis (a metabolic state in which the blood becomes too acidic) under these circumstances. Another potentially negative aspect of Glucophage, though, is the fact that it can erase ovulatory abnormalities found in some overweight girls who have gone through puberty, leading to a greater risk of unplanned pregnancies in sexually active teenagers taking it.

Long periods of high blood sugars should be avoided, so if adequate glycemic control is not achieved within three to six months on Glucophage alone, then additional therapies should be initiated. Many people with type 2 diabetes need more than one medication, and the preferred approach by physicians is to add another without withdrawing ones already being used. Other medications include those from the sulfonylurea class (such as Glynase or Glucotrol), which work by stimulating the pancreas to produce more insulin. Certain drugs in this class, such as DiaBeta and Micronase, have a longer duration of action and are more likely to cause low blood sugar—particularly when physical activity is initiated. Your child needs to frequently monitor his or her blood sugars when initiating more exercise if taking this medication.

Other possible additions include Prandin or Starlix, which may have advantages for teens who eat only sporadically as they can be taken specifically with meals to promote additional insulin release to cover glycemic responses to the food. As for insulin sensitizers, at least one drug from the thiazolidenedione class was taken off the market (Rezulin, which may cause liver damage), but Avandia and Actos are generally being prescribed for use by 10 percent or more of youth with type 2 diabetes without significant side effects. They improve insulin resistance (a major issue for these kids), do not cause hypoglycemia, and can be taken once daily. In adults, these medications have been found to occasionally cause fluid retention, but less so in youth.

The last class, alpha-glucosidase inhibitors, works by slowing the absorption of carbohydrates from the gut, but any advantages of their use by youth are not known at this time. However, a new class of diabetic medications known as incretins (a sixth class) is being investigated. Incretins appear to simultaneously stimulate the release of insulin, inhibit the liver's release of glucose (by blocking glucagon release), and delay the emptying of food from the stomach. One such drug in this class,

Exenatide, is currently undergoing clinical trials in adults and may be another choice for your child's treatment in the future.

If the blood glucose is quite high at diagnosis (greater than 250 mg/dl), medications may need to be initiated immediately, which may later be decreased or withdrawn if lifestyle changes are effective in achieving good blood sugar control. A recent study actually showed that when people newly diagnosed with type 2 diabetes are started on insulin immediately, good control is rapidly achieved. Doing so appears to have a positive residual effect, as these people are not likely to still need supplemental insulin a year later.

Insulin and the Like

To achieve good glycemic control, many kids with type 2 diabetes must take supplemental insulin injections. A wide variety of insulin and insulin analogs (modified insulins) are now available that can be used safely in diabetic youth. Once- or twice-a-day dosing can be done with some of the longer-acting choices, such as Lantus (an analog designed to cover basal insulin needs for twenty-four hours) or Detemir (the newest basal analog requiring two daily injections, twelve hours apart). Another choice of many physicians is NPH, an intermediate-acting insulin; some practitioners have diabetic youth combine daytime oral medications with an injection of NPH at bedtime to prevent elevated fasting blood sugars in the morning. Unfortunately, insulin use generally promotes weight gain, but combining daytime oral medications with nighttime NPH causes the least gain. Another combination option that has been used successfully once glycemia is under better control with insulin is to add in Glucophage and then slow or stop insulin use.

If glycemic control is not achieved with any of these longer-acting insulins alone, short-acting bolus insulins, such as Humalog, Novolog, or Regular, all exerting their main effects within one to three hours after injection, can also be prescribed for dosing with meals. In some cases, youth with type 2 diabetes are started on an insulin pump, which can be programmed to continuously deliver small basal doses of short-acting insulin (to mimic the coverage of the longer-acting options) along with bolus doses of the same to cover carbohydrate intake in meals and snacks.

In children who have many of the classic diabetic symptoms (excessive thirst, hunger, and/or urination) and greatly elevated blood sugars, treatment with insulin is strongly recommended (whether at bedtime only, twice daily, or multiple dosing). If symptoms persist or glycemia cannot be controlled well with or without insulin, testing urine for the presence of excessive ketones may be helpful to identify if your child actually has type 1 diabetes and not type 2. Type 1 diabetes invariably requires more frequent dosing of insulin to cover not only basal needs, but also meals and snacks. Remember to work with your child's healthcare team to learn how to make appropriate adjustments to his or her insulin doses.

Other Supplements for Diabetic Youth

Whether people need to take supplemental vitamins, minerals, and other compounds is currently being hotly debated in the nutritional world. While some experts claim that you can get everything your body needs by simply consuming a nutritionally balanced diet, many others loudly denounce these claims, instead asserting that nutritional supplements are absolutely required, especially for anyone with a chronic health condition like diabetes. While the jury is still out on the issue of supplementation, enough evidence is available that supports the belief that diabetes itself creates a special metabolic situation—particularly when blood sugars are not well controlled—that may cause your child's body to become more depleted of certain nutrients; likewise, such deficiencies may be improved with the addition of nutrient-filled foods or specific supplements. Among these are a variety of antioxidant vitamins and minerals, as well as magnesium, chromium, vanadium, and vitamin D. More information on which foods contain these nutrients can be easily accessed at www.nal.usda.gov/fnic/foodcomp, www.cc.nih.gov/ccc/supplements, and www.cfsan.fda.gov/~dms/supplmnt.html.

Before putting your diabetic child or the rest of the family on any of these supplements, remember that for any supplemental nutrients to be effective, you usually must be deficient in them, or else you are wasting your money. Being insulin resistant and hyperglycemic can, however, potentially cause certain nutrient deficiencies. If your child can control his or her diabetes with the dietary and physical activity changes suggested in this book, then supplements may not be additionally helpful, particularly because the effects of most nutrients are likely synergistic with other compounds found in whole foods. Simply encourage your kids to eat more foods in their natural state to obtain them.

Antioxidants

Hyperglycemia increases oxidative stress, which occurs when more oxygen "free radicals" are produced than your body can quench. Accumulated oxidative stress may ultimately result in many of the complications associated with long-term diabetes, including heart disease and eye, kidney, and nerve damage. High levels of blood sugar, elevated circulating insulin, and insulin resistance together enhance free radical production in people with type 2 diabetes, and these radical compounds then promote further insulin resistance and a lower insulin secretion—a veritable downhill spiral for insulin action.

If you have diabetes, why can't you quench all of these "radicals" on your own? Everyone's body possesses antioxidant enzyme systems that normally are able to fight free radicals; however, diabetes—particularly when poorly controlled—not only increases free radical generation, but at the same time also depresses the body's natural antioxidant defenses. Thus, diabetic people with high levels of oxidative stress and/or depletion of natural antioxidant defense systems are the most likely to benefit from antioxidant therapy. While certain diabetic medications (e.g., gliclazide, a sulfonylurea used outside of the United States) can potentially lower oxidative stress, antioxidant nutrients may be most effective in complementing or augmenting the body's own ability to combat these diabetes-related demons.

Specific dietary antioxidants appear to be of particular benefit in treating and preventing diabetes and its complications: Primary among these are vitamin E, glutathione, alpha lipoic acid, vitamin C, beta-carotene, selenium, copper, and zinc. In addition, CoQ_{10} (informally known as vitamin K) may also play a role in preventing oxidative stress. For example, diabetic cataract formation results, in part, from deficient glutathione levels, which contribute to a faulty antioxidant defense system within the lens of the eye; nutrients that increase glutathione and its activity include lipoic acid, vitamins E and C, and selenium. Take heed, though: In excessive (i.e., large supplemental) doses, almost all antioxidants have been shown to act as pro-oxidants, resulting in exactly the opposite of the desired effect.

On the other hand, it is impossible to overdose on antioxidants if they are obtained naturally through food, so it is far better to obtain them that way whenever possible. Some surprising consumables contain large amounts of various antioxidants. For example, a recent study found that a typical cup of hot cocoa (containing two tablespoons of pure cocoa powder) has twice as many of these health-promoting compounds (flavonoids in particular) as red wine, two to three times more than green tea, and four to five times more than black tea. Drinking it hot also apparently releases more antioxidant power, but all of us would do better to use the sugar-free variety.

Vitamin E

A family of "tocopherols," vitamin E is a fat-soluble vitamin that scavenges peroxyl radicals that damage cell membranes; by doing so, it effectively prevents the oxidation of unsaturated (good) fats in various membranes around the body, including those found in red blood cells, nerves, and lungs. This vitamin also reduces oxidative stress in the arteries, which has the potential to reduce plaque formation there, in part by making the bad cholesterol (LDL) less susceptible to oxidation and lowering its ability to accelerate heart disease. Unfortunately, most recent research has not shown that vitamin E supplementation effectively combats cardiovascular disease, and combining its intake with Lipitor (a cholesterol-lowering drug) may actually have detrimental effects.

Supplementation with vitamin E, though, may be effective in combating excessive oxidation of other fats, a major cause of diabetes-related tissue damage in eyes (cataract formation), nerves (tingling, numbness, and pain), muscles (weakness and atrophy), and immune cells (increased susceptibility to infections). Furthermore, low serum levels of vitamin E have even been associated with a greater risk of developing type 2 diabetes.

In foods, vitamin E can be found naturally in vegetable oils, seeds (especially sunflower), nuts (particularly almonds), green, leafy vegetables (like spinach and broccoli), margarine, fortified breakfast cereals, tomato products, sweet potatoes, and wheat germ. Unfortunately, cooking and food processing may destroy this vitamin in many foods, making it difficult to obtain adequately from the diet. Vitamin E supplements can be taken to correct any deficiencies. These capsules usually contain the alpha form of this vitamin, as opposed to the mix of forms found naturally in foods, however. For kids six to twelve years old, only 400 IU would be recommended as a daily supplement; for ages thirteen and up, as much as 800 IU is considered safe.

Glutathione and Alpha Lipoic Acid

Glutathione is the main antioxidant found in all cells. This substance and alpha lipoic acid (LA) are the two most important antioxidants in your body, and both are made by your body itself. Comprised of three amino acids found abundantly in foods, glutathione protects the DNA in cell nuclei from being oxidized. However, your body may not always synthesize enough to meet your need for it, but it can also be obtained from various vegetables and fruits, such as asparagus, avocados, spinach, strawberries, peaches, melons, and citrus fruits.

While lipoic acid increases glutathione levels by helping cells absorb a critical amino acid needed for its synthesis, LA also guards against common diabetic complications, including stroke, heart attacks, peripheral nerve damage, and cataracts, as well as memory loss, cancer, and aging effects. Spinach (raw or cooked) is the best source of this nutrient, which is also found naturally in small amounts in broccoli, tomatoes, potatoes, peas, and Brussels sprouts. In particular, spinach is touted for its ability to fight cataracts (common in people with diabetes) and macular degeneration (the leading cause of blindness in all adults).

For people with diabetes, these two natural antioxidants may be even more vital. Lipoic acid has been shown to have the ability to normalize diabetes-induced renal (kidney) dysfunction and to lower other biomarkers of oxidative stress, including potential damage to the nerve cells, where it additionally promotes nerve fiber regeneration and stimulates a substance known as nerve growth factor. Glutathione levels may be depleted by elevated blood glucose levels in various tissues around the body, which, in poorly controlled diabetes, leaves the door wide open for increased oxidative damage. In fact, the maintenance of normal levels of glutathione is of utmost importance in preventing diabetic cataracts. So, now is definitely the time to get your whole family to start eating spinach at least a couple of times a week.

Vitamin C

Also known as ascorbic acid, vitamin C is a water-soluble vitamin with strong antioxidant qualities. Think about what happens to a sliced apple when it sits on the counter: The exposed surfaces start to turn brown due to exposure to oxygen in the air, which oxidizes them. You can prevent this oxidation from occurring by coating the apple with lemon or orange juice, both of which are high in vitamin C.

While deficiencies of this vitamin are rare in the United States, serum levels of vitamin C have been found to be lower in some individuals with insulin resistance at high risk for developing type 2 diabetes. Moreover, although this vitamin is generally considered to be less effective in combating diabetic complications than vitamin E and other antioxidants, when supplemented by people with type 2 diabetes, it reduces blood pressure and improves the elasticity of the arterial walls—both of which reduce the risk of heart disease. A definite role for vitamin C in the prevention and treatment of diabetic eye diseases, including cataracts and glaucoma (the second leading cause of new blindness), has also been established, likely because oxidative stress is a major contributor to their development.

This vitamin is abundant in citrus fruits, bell peppers, peaches, strawberries, broccoli, and salad greens. The recommended intake of 200 mg per day can easily be obtained through food intake. Megadosing with supplemental vitamin C is controversial, though, as doses of 1,000 mg (1 gram) per day or more may contribute to the formation of kidney stones in susceptible people or result in rebound scurvy (a disease affecting collagen that vitamin C normally prevents) when supplements are stopped. Given these potential risks, vitamin C is best obtained naturally through your family's diet or through smaller supplemental doses (no more than 200 mg per day).

Beta-carotene

Beta-carotene, one compound in a family of carotenoids, may not be a first-line antioxidant in the body according to the latest research, but it does function as an antioxidant at some level. It has the capacity to boost the activity of tumor-scavenging, natural killer cells, which are an integral part of our cell-based immune system. Along with other antioxidants, it also helps inhibit cholesterol synthesis, facilitate cellular interactions, and stimulate enzymes that repair damaged DNA. This provitamin is also a significant source of vitamin A (your body converts beta-carotene to the active form of vitamin A, retinol, as needed), which plays a role in the health of the retina (the back of the eye often damaged by diabetes), immune system, skin, epithelial cells (they line the organs and are where cancers start), and memory.

Beta-carotene can be found naturally in greatest abundance in yellow-orange vegetables like carrots, pumpkin, squash, and sweet potatoes, as well as green, leafy vegetables (spinach, kale, turnip greens, and broccoli) and tomato products. Supplements are generally less effective than consuming this provitamin in its natural form, as foods also contain other carotenoids, including alpha-carotene, which may actually prove to be a more effective cancer fighter than the beta form. Megadoses are generally considered to be harmless, though—unlike excessive intake of vitamin A—but adequate amounts of beta-carotene can easily be obtained through a balanced diet.

Selenium

This trace mineral is thought to have antioxidant qualities, as it is essential for the proper functioning of one of the body's antioxidant enzymes, glutathione peroxidase, which specifically works to prevent damage to the membranes of our oxygen-carrying red blood cells (among others). It is believed to work in concert with vitamin E in this respect. Selenium may play an important role in the prevention of diabetic cataracts as well. Brazil nuts are a particularly good source of selenium (one nut contains a full day's requirements), but it can also be obtained through intake of most types of fish, poultry, and whole-grain products (at least in the United States, where the soil is selenium rich).

Copper

Among other things, this trace mineral is a component of another antioxidant enzyme called superoxide dismutase (SOD). Lower levels of this enzyme have been found in diabetic people with kidney disease. Copper deficiency due to inadequate dietary intake is not known to normally exist in humans, however. This nutrient can be found in beef, shellfish, baking chocolate, mushrooms, nuts (cashews, Brazil nuts, walnuts), sunflower seeds, legumes, potatoes, and couscous. Supplements are not recommended, though, as excessive copper intake via supplements can be toxic to the body.

Zinc

Another trace mineral, zinc is a component of over one hundred enzymes, many of which are involved in glucose metabolism. A mild dietary zinc deficiency is thought to be common in the United States, particularly if intake of animal protein is relatively low, given that it is mainly found in oysters and other shellfish, meats, and poultry, although lesser amounts are available in whole grains, dairy products, fortified breakfast cereals, semisweet chocolate, nuts, and seeds. Zinc lozenges are also widely available in drug and food stores as a potential treatment for the common cold, although it has not been definitively proven effective in this regard.

Diabetes apparently affects zinc status, though, potentially resulting in a deficiency when more of it is lost in the urine (and poorly controlled diabetes causes excessive urination). Since zinc plays a clear role in the synthesis, storage, and secretion of insulin from functional beta cells, a deficiency may interfere with the normal release of insulin in people with type 2 diabetes. Furthermore, several diabetic complications may be related to increased oxidative stress associated with decreases in zinc, as the function of the SOD enzyme (mentioned in relation to copper) is also dependent on the availability of adequate zinc.

Some practitioners may make a case for zinc supplementation, if a deficiency is determined to be present in your child. However, be forewarned that supplements containing even 25 mg per day (the recommended intake is 15 mg for adults) may interfere with the absorption of other minerals, such as copper and iron, even though the upper intake level for zinc via supplements is currently set at 40 mg daily. Doses over 100 mg daily may actually increase the "bad" cholesterol in your blood while lowering the "good" type, as well as contributing to the development of anemia. Therefore, only a low-dose supplement would be advisable if adequate zinc cannot be taken in through dietary changes.

Magnesium

The fourth most abundant mineral found in the body, magnesium is widely distributed in foods, particularly in nuts (Brazil nuts, almonds, and cashews, for example), seafood, leafy green vegetables (spinach), other fruits and vegetables (including bananas), whole-grain products, oat bran, semisweet chocolate, and legumes. This mineral affects bone health and, in muscles, it is an integral component of over 300 enzymes, most of which affect your metabolism. It also helps control blood pressure, regulate the rhythm of your heart, prevent muscle cramps, and improve the action of insulin in the body.

Accordingly, low levels of magnesium have been associated with both increased blood pressure and type 2 diabetes. In fact, low serum levels have been found to be a strong, independent predictor of diabetes, likely because magnesium facilitates the action of insulin and aids enzymes involved in carbohydrate metabolism; thus, a magnesium deficiency may interfere with the binding of insulin, uptake of glucose into cells, and glucose use. In fact, a recent, well-designed study confirmed that 2.5 grams of a magnesium chloride solution taken daily for sixteen weeks improves insulin sensitivity and glycemic control in older people with type 2 diabetes with previously low levels of serum magnesium.

In people free of diabetes, magnesium levels are not normally low; however, this mineral, like zinc, can be depleted through excessive urination resulting from poorly controlled diabetes. Sweating also increases losses of this mineral, so regular sports participation may increase dietary needs. On the other hand, too much magnesium can cause transient diarrhea, but is otherwise considered safe. The main exception is in people with kidney failure, whose magnesium intake must be restricted.

If your child's diabetes control is less than optimal, you may want to assess his or her current dietary magnesium intake before deciding to supplement. Muscle cramps may be one symptom of a deficiency. Adults should generally not supplement with more than 350 mg daily; however, higher levels in adults have been taken with minimal side effects. If your child's blood sugars are well controlled, he or she will not likely need to take supplemental magnesium, though. Instead, increase your family's intake with healthier food choices, since it is available in such a wide variety of foods.

Chromium

Chromium enhances the activity of insulin by increasing the binding of insulin to receptors in fat and muscle, as well as the total number of insulin receptors and their activity. While deficiencies of this mineral in a normal population are rare, supplements given to people with diabetes can improve their glucose tolerance, along with their antioxidant enzyme status, when given alone or in combination with zinc. When blood sugar levels are normal, extra intake of chromium has minimal effects, but when chronic hyperglycemia is present, this mineral may help reduce blood glucose levels by improving insulin action.

This trace mineral can be obtained through intake of meat, organ meats, oysters (a particularly good source), cheese, whole-grain products, asparagus, and beer (not by the kids, though!). If you decide to use a chromium supplement, doses of less than 1,000 micrograms per day appear safe for short-term use by adults, but should not exceed 200 micrograms per day when taken long term. Safe, supplemental doses for children have not been determined, but should likely not exceed 200 micrograms daily.

Vanadium and Vanadyl Salts

When taken as vanadyl sulfate, as a salt of vanadium, this trace mineral, which is considered a nonessential nutrient, has recently been found to exert a glucose-lowering effect in people with diabetes by decreasing the liver's production of glucose, along with increasing the insulin sensitivity of muscles. Through these actions, vanadyl ions may be effective not only in treating or relieving diabetes, but also in preventing its onset. Treatment with vanadyl sulfate has also been shown to increase glutathione levels in the kidneys of diabetic rats, and, therefore, it may also be effective in preventing renal diabetic complications.

Good food sources of vanadium include shellfish, whole-grain products, parsley, mushrooms, and black pepper. The average American diet supplies 15 to 30 micrograms of vanadium daily, but since it has not been deemed "essential" in the diet, no recommended intake has been established. When supplements are taken in larger doses, though, diarrhea can result, and the safety of such doses has yet to be determined. Thus, you would be best advised to consult with your health-care provider before starting your family on vanadium supplements of any sort.

Vitamin D

This fat-soluble vitamin is best known for its hormonelike role in increasing the body's absorption of dietary calcium and, thus, promoting bone health. Particularly during the winter, a vitamin D deficiency may partly contribute to impairments in insulin secretion and action. In fact, new evidence now suggests that low vitamin D status is a risk factor for type 2 diabetes and prediabetes, as a deficiency worsens pancreatic beta cell function. The biologically active form of vitamin D is also a potent modulator of the immune system and, as such, is thought to potentially act to prevent the development of autoimmune-based type 1 diabetes.

Most foods do not naturally contain any of this vitamin, but it can be obtained through fortified dairy products, margarine, and fish oils.

One glass of vitamin D fortified milk will provide 25 percent of the daily requirements for a child, so if your kids drink soda instead of low-fat milk, they may not be getting enough. You can also obtain this vitamin through exposure to sunlight, during which the UVB rays convert vitamin D_3, a prohormone, into the active form of this vitamin, calcitriol. In order for this conversion to occur, you must expose at least your hands, arms, and face to sunlight for ten to twenty minutes during the summer, two to three times per week. Longer exposure is needed for the same effect during the winter, and consequently, many people are somewhat deficient in this vitamin during those months, especially if they live in northern latitudes. In the absence of adequate sunlight, supplementation of up to 200 IU, or 5 micrograms, for children and adults is prudent. However, this vitamin is potentially toxic in large doses, so supplementation beyond the recommended daily levels is not advised.

If your child is not successful in controlling his or her blood sugars with the first two cornerstones of diabetes management—diet and exercise—alone, please don't feel that you have somehow failed as a parent. Diabetes is a progressive disease in adults and likely also in kids, although its reversal in youth is more possible. The key to preventing diabetic complications, though, is undeniably optimizing blood sugar control. Focus on your child's blood sugars through whatever means possible, even if that includes a diabetic medication or two or even supplemental insulin.

So, what's the bottom line on supplements, then? Reading through all of the information on such nutrients can admittedly be overwhelming. The best recommendation for improving your family's nutrient intake is to first make the dietary changes recommended earlier in this book. Next, make certain that you have added in key foods high in antioxidants and other potentially diabetes-depleted nutrients, including spinach, broccoli, and other leafy dark green vegetables, nuts and seeds, sweet potatoes (without adding extra sugar, though), whole grains, tomatoes, strawberries, peaches, citrus fruits, black pepper, and even limited amounts of semisweet chocolate, the darker the better. If you can get your family eating more of these foods and fewer highly refined ones, as an added bonus, their insulin sensitivity will improve.

CONCLUSION

A FTER MAKING it to the final section of this book, your head may be filled with what feels like an overabundance of new and useful ideas and knowledge, or maybe you feel like it all made sense when you read it, but now you cannot remember a single thing. In either case, follow the KISS principle, and you will at least emerge with enough information to keep your prediabetic child from developing diabetes, improve his or her current state of insulin resistance and body weight, or control elevated blood sugar levels more effectively if already diagnosed with type 2 diabetes. This principle is commonly referred to as the "Keep It Simple, Stupid" approach, although some may argue that the last "S" should stand for "and Systematic" instead for best results.

Follow the Basics

To prevent and control type 2 diabetes in youth, then, let's not lose the forest in the trees. Rather than focus solely on individual, pragmatic solutions, we need to also focus on societal problems as causes of obesity, prediabetes, and type 2 diabetes in our youth and how to fix them. "Simple" is good because with human nature being the way it is, if a solution is too difficult or too confusing, we will choose not do it. "Systematic" is also practical because the definition of a "system" is "a group of interacting elements functioning as a complex whole." We must first understand the underlying cause of a problem and then devise solutions that address its origins. In essence, we need to focus, individually and as a society, on solving the problem of the two types of chips mentioned earlier: potato chips and computer chips.

Anti-chip Activities

Potato chips by themselves are not inherently evil (when eaten in moderation), but they do succinctly exemplify the first major problem with our youth: overconsumption of nutritionally poor foods. Access to a plethora of calorie-dense, nutrient-poor foods equates to a nutritional nightmare for our children and society as a whole.

The second problem is that our children are undeniably too sedentary. Why? The second type of chips, computer chips, is causing us all to be physically inactive. Although time-saving devices, computers, cell phones, PDAs, and other advanced technologies allow us to get more work done in less time, they also take away much of our movement. Almost invariably, children will remain glued to any type of screen they can find (TV, computer, video game, etc.) for hours on end, if you let them.

Now that we know what really causes insulin resistance and the majority of the cases of type 2 diabetes in kids, it makes sense for us to act as physicians do, by attempting to standardize the key elements of care to solve the problem. As parents and caregivers, we desperately need to speak out to keep physical education programs in our schools and fast-food vendors out. We also have to make a commitment on a more personal level to enable our kids to participate in extracurricular sports and active leisure pursuits—or just being more physically active however and whenever they can.

What can you do? Well, for starters, brush off all of your bikes in the garage, pump up their tires, and go out for a family bike ride. Also, painful though it may be for all concerned, be committed to setting time limits for TV watching and sedentary video or computer game playing and actually *enforcing* them (two hours a day maximum is advisable). Set daily, weekly, monthly, and yearly exercise goals for your family, and whenever they have a free moment, get your kids to do something active. Then, take a look at the foods your family is eating in and out of your home and start to make changes—small ones that equate to a larger overall effect are sufficient. As a start, just cutting out all regular soft drinks and other sugary fluids will help, as well as limiting your family's consumption of refined "white" foods. Your ultimate goal is to get back to the basics by trying to eat more natural foods, particularly those with a lower glycemic effect.

Simple Steps to a Healthier Lifestyle

Lifestyle changes are important in forming optimal nutritional and exercise habits for lifelong good health, not just for weight loss. You also want to make changes that are sustainable in the long run—that is, permanent. It is never too late to teach an old dog new tricks, but doing so is certainly easier when we start our kids off young in learning a healthier way to live.

We need to promote a healthy lifestyle to our kids in a way that they can understand. First, we have to be good role models. Parents who want healthy lives for their children must first adopt them for themselves—including not only optimal nutrition, but also daily physical activity and a positive attitude about themselves and their bodies. If you are obsessed with your own body weight and shape, then your children will adopt the same attitude about themselves.

Along the same lines, never make an issue out of a child's body weight. Don't label kids as "chubby" or "fat." Everyone's shape is different, and your child may or may not be shaped just like you. If your children are different from each other, do not treat the heavier ones differently with regard to what foods they are allowed to eat. The whole family should be eating the same healthy foods, so change everyone's diet together for the better. Also, remember to never use food as a reward or withhold it as a punishment. Even more importantly, do not put young kids on low-calorie diets as they can be nutritionally deficient; instead, modify a growing child's portions and choose healthier selections. In addition, emphasize eating a variety of foods to make sure that your kids are getting all of the vitamins, minerals, and phytonutrients that they need for good health.

You can even involve your children in creating small, achievable goals on their way to a healthier lifestyle. Talk about recommended servings from the food groups and find out which foods they like that fall into the various categories. For younger kids, you might have them pick a color to represent the foods they eat every day (e.g., green for veggies, red for fruits, white for dairy, etc.). By the end of each day, you can help them make sure that they have eaten all of these foods. Older kids may enjoy tracking their food intake along with their moods and activity levels. It may help them realize why they eat—out of boredom, anger, or depression, to procrastinate from doing their homework, or just because they eat mindlessly while watching TV.

Make Good Health a Family Affair

Another key to a healthier lifestyle is to involve the whole family in any major adjustments. The best compliance by the kids happens when at least one parent partakes in the same lifestyle changes, and the results are even better when a complete diet and exercise overhaul happens for everyone in the family at the same time.

Include the Whole Family

When I was diagnosed with diabetes (type 1) as a very young child, my biggest disappointment was that I had to give up my favorite cereal back then, Froot Loops. At that time, my mother wisely made the decision that in order for me to comply with the dietary recommendations for diabetes management at the time with the least amount of emotional distress, she would not only change my diet, but also the whole family's diet to coincide with mine. The result? My older brother had to give up Froot Loops, too, and we all gained an undeniably healthier diet in the process.

Back when I began living with diabetes in the late 1960s, there were no blood glucose meters to use at home and no other form of instantaneous feedback about blood sugar control other than the way I felt. As a result of my early experiences with diabetes, to this day (despite now having a blood glucose meter at my disposal and a vial of quick-acting insulin) I can attest to the fact that the glycemic effect of many foods makes a difference not only in my blood glucose control, but also how I physically feel. Thus, by choice, I still avoid certain foods, such as Froot Loops and other sugared breakfast cereals, breakfast bars, cake, pastries, and most candy, all of which cause a rapid spike in my blood sugar. Why? Because I find that even with the option of giving an injection of rapid-acting insulin to cover such carbohydrates, it is still difficult for insulin to keep up with foods that cause large glycemic spikes. When my blood sugars invariably shoot up after eating such foods, I instantly begin to feel bad in a physical sense—sluggish, lethargic, hungry (not a true stomach "growling," but rather a drive to eat despite being full), and sleepy. Sometimes my head even begins to hurt.

Similar symptoms will very likely result in a type 2 diabetic child who eats a poor diet. Although his or her circulating insulin may still be abundant, keep in mind that type 2 diabetes resulted when the beta cells were no longer able to keep up with your child's exorbitantly high insulin needs. Eating higher-GI/GL foods will overload his or her body with glucose and cause your child to feel equally bad, even if he or she is not as acutely aware of these symptoms as I am by being completely dependent on injected insulin.

So, knowing the consequences, why do people continue to eat unhealthily? Merely providing information about diet and exercise and emphasizing their importance in everyday life is apparently not sufficient to cause the widespread lifestyle changes that Americans in particular desperately need. Despite the potential for health improvements in a variety of susceptible populations—including people with diabetes and others with heart disease, insulin resistance, high blood pressure, and poor nutrition—studies have shown that most people who have succeeded in making positive lifestyle changes have needed an active, assertive program of individualized guidance and supervision.

Nevertheless, the chances of succeeding on your own are better when change is a family affair. Why is family support of lifestyle changes so important? A cynic might say it is because misery loves company, but those of us who have implemented such changes already know that they have made us anything but miserable. On the contrary, good health resulting from a healthy lifestyle is a precious commodity that money truly cannot buy. We all need emotional support to implement lifestyle changes, though. Imagine how difficult it would be to get your kids to stop eating doughnuts if, against your wishes, your husband brought them home for the family on a regular basis. Instead, if the whole family agreed to moderately limit doughnut consumption to once a month (rather than completely abstaining), then such a change would be more successfully achieved. Meeting up with a friend or group for walks or workouts increases the likelihood that you will do them as well—even if you only show up to keep other people from nagging you about slouching. You can even have family meetings to plan out increased physical activity and decreased inactivity and set goals.

Tips for Making Healthy Lifestyle Changes a Family Affair

•

- Pay attention to your own attitudes and behaviors toward your body weight, food, and physical activity first
- Enlist total family involvement and form a positive support system for changes
- Get back to basics as soon as possible by including more basic and natural foods in your family's diet
- Eat the same foods and exercise together so healthier living is not regarded as an isolated punishment for heavier members of the family
- Eliminate all practices that encourage overeating in your household, such as forcing your kids to "clean their plates"
- Never use food as a reward for good behavior or exercise
- Help your kids identify and change inappropriate food habits, such as snacking on high-calorie foods while watching TV
- Involve your children in preparing healthier meals and snacks for the family
- Start the whole family keeping a food and activity log to chart progress and goals
- Make meals a pleasant family experience; turn the TV off, eat slowly, enjoy your food, converse with one another, and get reacquainted
- Avoid "family style" meals where everyone digs into a large platter of food; instead, portion out appropriate amounts of food for your kids
- Implement a fifteen-minute waiting period for second helpings for everyone to allow their stomach enough time to signal its fullness to the brain
- Make being physically active fun for everyone by including family bike rides, backyard Frisbee games, hiking trips, or just dancing around the living room
- Know your respective roles: Parents should establish some controls and limits, such as proper portions at meals, but children can make

some age-appropriate decisions for themselves, such as which activity to do on a given day

• Keep in mind that the goal of your lifestyle improvements is not really weight loss per se, but rather the adoption of healthy habits to prevent further weight gain

Include Other Important Players

If you can, also involve your children's teachers, coaches, and other adults in implementing these positive lifestyle changes. Many kids interact with other adults much more than they do with their own parents, and young children in particular look up to their teachers as role models. Many teachers also need to be reminded not to use candy and unhealthy food for rewards for good grades and student behavior. The same applies to coaches of soccer and other extracurricular sports teams. Positive behaviors and accomplishments always should be reinforced with praise and love, not sugary treats.

For the best chance of success, your "extended family" should include your child's health-care providers as well. A major cause of noncompliance with diabetes treatment plans (including lifestyle changes) is poor communication between doctors and their patients. Researchers have found that people with diabetes often receive incomplete or conflicting information about their condition and its treatment from their physicians. Many patients also report not feeling any different whether or not they adhered to recommended treatments, showing that their health beliefs may also negatively impact compliance. When diabetes health-care providers meet regularly with patients and provide them with simple flowcharts for their care, they take their oral diabetic medications more regularly and blood sugar control improves.

Get Started

It has been said that the definition of insanity is repeating the same behavior and expecting different results. I am not asking you to necessarily dramatically change your family's lifestyle, but prevention and control of obesity and type 2 diabetes in your kids is going to involve doing something differently, permanently. The healthy lifestyle changes that you implement now for yourself and your family are not the same as "going on a diet," which implies that the "diet" will end at some point. Instead, you are simply converting to a new plan for healthier living. If you avoid calling your meal plan a "diet," everyone will have a much more positive attitude toward the changes you implement. Along the same lines, if "exercise" is a four-letter word around your household, just consider your kids as becoming more "physically active" throughout the day, and try to get them to sit less and move more.

If some degree of weight loss is your family's goal, do yourselves a favor and do *not* follow any drastic fad diet or unbalanced diet plans. Remember, prepubescent children really should not be placed on any diet due to its potential to deprive them of nutrients needed for growth. Also, teens really should avoid dieting since they are at the age when most eating disorders develop, and most start with dieting. We adults may need to lose a few pounds (or more), but since most diets fail, we will likely gain the weight back afterward anyway—unless we adopt a healthy eating plan and incorporate more physical activity into our lives, that is. It's time for your whole family to give up dieting, develop a healthy relationship with eating in general, start moving more, and take it one day at a time.

Finally ready to begin taking steps to improve your family's health? Great! Now is the time to get up, start moving, and put your family's healthier lifestyle into high gear. See you and your kids out at the park and in the produce section at the grocery store.

APPENDIX A:
GENERAL FOOD SHOPPING GUIDE

Consume More of	Use Very Occasionally	Try to Avoid Altogether
Water; noncaloric drinks; diet, non-cola, caffeine-free soda	Diet, caffeinated sodas; regular iced tea; sports drinks	Regular sodas, especially colas; sugary, noncarbonated drinks
Fresh, raw vegetables; plain, frozen vegetables	Vegetables grilled in oil or butter; highly salted vegetables; processed tomato sauces	Canned vegetables; vegetables with added sauces (cream, butter); battered, fried vegetables
Whole fruits; dried fruits (in small portions); canned fruits in natural juices (drained)	100% fruit juices (except apple and white grape); dried fruits with added sweeteners	Fruit "drinks" and "cocktails"; apple and white grape juices; canned fruits in heavy syrup

Consume More of	Use Very Occasionally	Try to Avoid Altogether
Whole-grain products (brown rice, oats, barley, etc.); sweet potatoes	Whole-wheat products (bread, crackers, bagels, pasta)	White-flour products (most crackers, doughnuts, breads, cakes, pastries, cookies); white potatoes
Products with no added sugars (and no unhealthy fats)	Products with small amounts of added sugars	Products with large amounts of added sugars
Old-fashioned oatmeal; high-fiber, low-sugar cereals	Quick oats with added sugar; cereals with moderate sugar	Highly processed breakfast cereals full of added sugar
Low-glycemic-index and -load carbohydrates	Moderate-glycemic-index and -load carbohydrates	High-glycemic-index and -load carbohydrates
Unsalted nuts; olive oil; canola oil; monounsaturated fat; liquid vegetable oils; cold-water fish	Salted nuts; reduced-fat margarine; polyunsaturated fat	Saturated fat; trans fat; butter or margarine; hydrogenated or partially hydrogenated oils
Nonfat, skim milk, ½%, or 1% dairy products	Low-fat (2%) or part skim dairy products	Whole-milk dairy products; cream
Ground turkey breast; skinless chicken and turkey breast; fish (not breaded or fried); legumes	Lean cuts of beef and pork; nonfat hot dogs and lunchmeat; turkey bacon; breaded, baked chicken breast (e.g., nuggets)	Steak; ground hamburger; bacon; sausage; hot dogs; regular lunchmeat; fatty cuts of beef and pork; fried chicken (breaded or skin on)
Steamed, broiled, or baked foods	Foods grilled in oil, butter, or margarine	Fried foods
Dark, semisweet chocolate	Regular chocolate; peanut M&M's; sugar-free candies	Sugary hard or other candy; Fruit Roll-Ups; Froot Snacks

APPENDIX B:
DIABETIC EXCHANGE DIET LISTS

THE FOLLOWING LISTS represent a more detailed presentation of the diabetic exchange diet discussed in chapter 2. Throughout, foods high in fiber (containing 3 grams or more per exchange serving) are marked with "☺" to indicate that these choices are healthier choices for your family, and items high in sodium (400 mg or more) are indicated by "☒" to remind you to limit your intake of them.

Carbohydrate, Protein, Fat, and Calories in One Serving from Each Exchange List

	Carbohydrate (grams)	Protein (grams)	Fat (grams)	Calories
1. Starch/Bread	15	3	trace	80
2. Meat				
Very lean	.	7	0–1	35
Lean	.	7	3	55
Medium-fat	.	7	5	75
High-Fat	.	7	8	100
3. Vegetable	5	2	.	25
4. Fruit	15	.	.	60
5. Milk				
Skim	12	8	0–3	90
Low-fat	12	8	5	120
Whole	12	8	8	150
6. Fat	.	.	5	45

I. Starch/Bread List

Each item in this list contains about 15 grams of carbohydrate, 3 grams of protein, a trace of fat, and 80 calories. Whole-grain products average about 2 grams of fiber per serving, but some are higher. Those foods that contain 3 or more grams of fiber per serving are marked with "☺." You can choose your starch exchanges from any of the items on this list. If you want to eat a starch food that is not on the list, the general rule is that ½ cup of cereal, grain, or pasta equals one serving, as does 1 ounce of a bread product.

Cereals/Grains/Pasta

☺ Bran cereals, concentrated (such as Bran Buds, All-Bran)	⅓ cup
☺ Bran cereals, flaked	½ cup
Bulgur (cooked)	½ cup
Cooked cereals	½ cup
Cornmeal (dry)	2½ Tbsp
Grape-Nuts	3 Tbsp
Grits (cooked)	½ cup
Other ready-to-eat, unsweetened (plain) cereals	¾ cup
Pasta (cooked)	½ cup
Puffed cereal	1½ cups
Rice, white or brown (cooked)	⅓ cup
Shredded wheat	½ cup
☺ Wheat germ	3 Tbsp

Dried Beans/Peas/Lentils

☺ Beans and peas (cooked) (such as kidney, white, split, blackeye)	⅓ cup
☺ Lentils (cooked)	⅓ cup
☺ Baked beans	¼ cup

Starchy Vegetables

☺ Corn	½ cup
☺ Corn on the cob, 6 inches	1 long
☺ Lima beans	½ cup
☺ Peas, green (canned or frozen)	½ cup
☺ Plaintain	½ cup
Potato, baked 1 small	(3 oz)
Potato, mashed	½ cup
Squash, winter (acorn, butternut)	¾ cup
Yam, sweet potato	⅓ cup

Bread

Bagel, ½	(1 oz)
Bread sticks, crisp, 4 inches long x ½ inch	2 (⅔ oz)
Croutons, low-fat	1 cup
English muffin	½
Frankfurter or hamburger bun	½ (1 oz)
Pita, 6 inches across	½
Plain roll, small	1 (1 oz)
Raisin, unfrosted	1 slice
☺ Rye, pumpernickel	1 slice (1 oz)
White (including French, Italian)	1 slice (1 oz)
Whole-wheat	1 slice

Crackers/Snacks

Animal crackers	8
Graham crackers, 2½-inch square	3
Matzoh	¾ oz
Melba toast	5 slices
Oyster crackers	24
Popcorn (popped, no fat added)	3 cups
Pretzels	¾ oz
Rye crisp (2 inches x 3½ inches)	4
Saltine-type crackers	6
Whole-wheat crackers, no fat added (crisp breads like Finn, Kavli, Wasa)	2–4 slices (¾ oz)

Starchy Foods Prepared with Added Fat
(count as 1 starch/bread serving, plus 1 fat serving)

Biscuit, 2½ inches across	1
Chow mein noodles	½ cup
Corn bread, 2-inch cube	1 (2 oz)
Cracker, round butter type	6
French-fried potatoes (2 inches to 3½ inches long)	10 (1½ oz)
Muffin, plain, small	1
Pancake, 4 inches across	2
Stuffing, bread (prepared)	¼ cup
Taco shell, 6 inches across	2
Waffle, 4½-inch square	1
Whole-wheat crackers, fat added (such as Triscuits)	4–6 (1 oz)

II. Meat List

Each serving of meat and substitutes on this list contains 7 grams of protein, but both the amount of fat and the calories vary with the kind of meat chosen. The list is divided into four parts, based on the amount of fat and calories: very lean meat, lean meat, medium-fat meat, and high-fat meat.

You are encouraged to use more lean and medium-fat meat, poultry, and fish in your meal plan in place of the high-fat selections to decrease your fat intake. Items in the high-fat group are high in saturated fat, cholesterol, and calories and should be limited as much as possible (no more than three times per week). Keep in mind that meat and substitutes do not contribute any fiber to your meal plan and many contain 400 mg or more of sodium per exchange ($\boxtimes$).

Lean Meat and Substitutes		
Beef	USDA Good or Choice grades of lean beef, such as round, sirloin, and flank steak; tenderloin; and chipped beef $\boxtimes$	1 oz
Pork	Lean pork, such as fresh ham; canned, cured, or boiled ham $\boxtimes$; Canadian bacon $\boxtimes$; tenderloin	1 oz
Veal	All cuts are lean except for veal cutlets (ground or cubed)	1 oz
Poultry	Chicken, turkey, Cornish hen (without skin)	1 oz
Fish	All fresh and frozen fish	1 oz
	Crab, lobster, scallops, shrimp, clams (fresh or canned in water $\boxtimes$)	2 oz
	Oysters	6 med
	Tuna $\boxtimes$ (canned in water)	¼ cup
	Herring (uncreamed or smoked)	1 oz
	Sardines (canned)	2 med
Wild game	Venison, rabbit, squirrel	1 oz
	Pheasant, duck, goose (without skin)	1 oz

Cheese	Any cottage cheese	¼ cup
	Grated parmesan	2 Tbsp
	Diet cheese ⊠ (with fewer than 55 calories per ounce)	1 oz
Other	95 percent fat-free luncheon meat	1 oz
	Egg whites	3
	Egg substitutes (with fewer than 55 calories per ¼ cup)	¼ cup

Medium-Fat Meat and Substitutes

Beef	Most beef products fall into this category. Examples are: all ground beef, roast (rib, chuck, rump), steak (cubed, Porterhouse, T-bone), and meat loaf	1 oz
Pork	Most pork products fall into this category (examples: chops, loin roast, Boston butt, cutlets)	1 oz
Lamb	Most lamb products fall into this category (examples: chops, leg, roast)	1 oz
Veal	Cutlet (ground or cubed, unbreaded)	1 oz
Poultry	Chicken (with skin), domestic duck or goose (well drained of fat), ground turkey	1 oz
Fish	Tuna ⊠ (canned in oil and drained)	¼ cup
	Salmon ⊠ (canned)	¼ cup
Cheese	Skim or part-skim milk cheeses, such as:	
	Ricotta	¼ cup
	Mozzarella	1 oz
	Diet cheeses ⊠ (with 56–80 calories per ounce)	1 oz
Other	86% fat-free luncheon meat ⊠	1 oz
	Egg (high in cholesterol, so limit to 3 per week)	1
	Egg substitutes (with 56–80 calories per ¼ cup)	¼ cup
	Tofu (2½ inch x 2¾ inch x 1 inch)	4 oz
	Liver, heart, kidney, sweetbreads (high in cholesterol)	1 oz

High-Fat Meat and Substitutes

Beef	Most USDA Prime cuts of beef, such as ribs, corned beef	1 oz
Pork	Spareribs, ground pork, pork sausage (patty or link)	1 oz
Lamb	Patties (ground lamb)	1 oz
Fish	Any fried fish product	1 oz
Cheese	All regular cheese ☒, such as American, blue, cheddar, Monterey, Swiss	1 oz
Other	Luncheon meat ☒, such as bologna, salami, pimiento loaf	1 oz
	Sausage ☒, such as Polish, Italian	1 oz
	Knockwurst, smoked	1 oz
	Bratwurst ☒	1 oz
	Frankfurter ☒ (turkey or chicken) (10/lb)	1 frank
	Peanut butter (contains unsaturated fat)	1 Tbsp

Meats That Count as One High-Fat Meat Plus One Fat Exchange

Frankfurter ☒	Beef, pork, or combo (400 mg or more of sodium per exchange) (10/lb)	1 frank

Additional Tips to Reduce Fat Intake

1. Bake, roast, broil, grill, or boil these foods rather than frying them with added fat.
2. Use a nonstick pan spray or a nonstick pan to brown or fry these foods.
3. Trim off visible fat before and after cooking.
4. Do not add flour, bread crumbs, coating mixes, or fat to these foods during cooking.
5. Weigh meat after removing bones and fat and again after cooking. Three ounces of cooked meat is equal to about 4 ounces of raw meat. Some examples of protein portions are the following: 2 ounces meat (2 meat exchanges) = 1 small chicken leg or thigh, ½ cup cottage cheese or tuna; 3 ounces meat (3 meat exchanges) = 1 medium pork chop, 1 small hamburger, ½ of a whole chicken breast, 1 unbreaded fish fillet, or cooked meat about the size of a deck of cards.

6. Restaurants usually serve prime cuts of meat, which are high in fat and calories.

III. Vegetable List

Each vegetable serving on this list contains about 5 grams of carbohydrate, 2 grams of protein, and 25 calories. Vegetables generally contain 2 to 3 grams of dietary fiber. Vegetables are a good source of vitamins and minerals, but fresh and frozen vegetables have more vitamins and less added salt than canned. However, rinsing canned vegetables will remove much of the salt. Starchy vegetables such as corn, peas, and potatoes are found on the Starch/Bread list, and "free" vegetables (i.e., fewer than 10 calories per serving) are in the Free Food list that follows.

Unless otherwise noted, the serving size for vegetables (one exchange) is ½ cup of cooked vegetables or vegetable juice or 1 cup of raw vegetables.

Fresh, Cooked, and Canned Vegetables	
Artichoke (½ medium)	Mushrooms, cooked
Asparagus	Okra
Beans (green, wax, Italian)	Onions
Bean sprouts	Pea pods
Beets	Peppers (green)
Broccoli	Rutabaga
Brussels sprouts	Sauerkraut
Cabbage, cooked	Spinach, cooked
Carrots	Summer squash (crookneck)
Cauliflower	Tomato (one large)
Eggplant	Tomato/vegetable juice
Greens (collard, mustard, turnip)	Turnips
Kohlrabi	Water chestnuts
Leeks	Zucchini, cooked

IV. Fruit List

Each item on this list contains about 15 grams of carbohydrate and 60 calories (each gram contains 4 calories). Fresh, frozen, and dried fruits have about 2 grams of fiber per serving, but some contain more. Fruit juices, however, contain very little dietary fiber. The carbohydrate and calorie contents for a fruit serving are based on the usual serving of the most commonly eaten fruits. Always use fresh, frozen, or canned fruits with no added sugar. Whole fruit is more filling than fruit juice and may be a better choice for those who are trying to lose weight or control blood sugars. Unless otherwise noted, the serving size for one fruit serving is ½ cup of fresh fruit or fruit juice and ¼ cup dried fruit.

Fresh, Frozen, and Unsweetened Canned Fruit	
Apples (raw, 2 inches across)	1
Applesauce (unsweetened)	½ cup
Apricots (raw or canned) (4 halves)	½ cup
Banana (9 inches long)	½
Blackberries (raw)	¾ cup
☺ Blueberries (raw)	¾ cup
Cantaloupe (5 inches across)	⅓ cup
Cantaloupe (cubes)	1 cup
Cherries (large, raw)	12 whole
Cherries (canned)	½ cup
Figs (raw, 2 inches across)	2
Fruit cocktail (canned)	½ cup
Grapefruit (medium)	½
Grapefruit (segments)	¾ cup
Grapes (small)	15
Honeydew melon (medium)	⅜
Honeydew melon (cubes)	1 cup

Kiwi (large)	1
Mandarin oranges	¾ cup
Mango (small)	½
Nectarines (2½ inches across)	1
Orange (2½ inches across)	1
Papaya	1 cup
Peach (2¾ inches across)	1
Peaches (canned) (2 halves)	1 cup
Pear (½ large)	1 small
Pears (canned) (2 halves)	½ cup
Persimmon (medium, native)	2
Pineapple (raw)	¾ cup
Pineapple (canned)	⅓ cup
Plum (raw, 2 inches across)	2
☺ Pomegranate	½
☺ Raspberries (raw)	1 cup
☺ Strawberries (raw, whole)	1¼ cups
Tangerine (2½ inches across)	2
Watermelon (cubes)	1¼ cups

☺ Dried Fruit

☺ Apples	4 rings
☺ Apricots	7 halves
Dates (medium)	2½
☺ Figs	1½
☺ Prunes (medium)	3
Raisins	2 Tbsp

Fruit Juice	
Apple juice/cider	½ cup
Cranberry juice cocktail	⅓ cup
Grapefruit juice	½ cup
Grape juice	⅓ cup
Orange juice	½ cup
Pineapple juice	½ cup
Prune juice	⅓ cup

V. Milk List

Each serving of milk or milk products on this list contains about 12 grams of carbohydrate and 8 grams of protein. The amount of fat in milk is measured in percent of butterfat, and calories vary with the kind of milk product chosen.

Dairy products (like milk, yogurt, and cheese) are the body's main source of calcium, but certainly not the only possible source. The whole-milk group has much more fat per serving than the other two groups; try to limit your choices from the whole-milk group as much as possible. Yogurt and many powdered milk products also have different amounts of fat, so read food labels to find out the fat and calorie content. Milk can be drunk or added to cereal or other foods. Also, many foods, such as sugar-free pudding, are made with milk (see the Combination Foods list that follows).

Skim and Very Low Fat Milk

Skim milk	1 cup
½% milk	1 cup
1% milk	1 cup
Low-fat buttermilk	1 cup
Evaporated skim milk	½ cup
Dry nonfat milk	⅓ cup
Plain nonfat yogurt	8 oz

Low-Fat Milk

2% milk	1 cup
Plain low-fat yogurt (with added nonfat milk solids)	8 oz

Whole Milk

Whole milk	1 cup
Evaporated whole milk	½ cup
Whole-milk plain yogurt	8 oz

VI. Fat List

Each serving on the fat list contains about 5 grams of fat and 45 calories. The foods on the fat list contain mostly fat, although some items may also contain a small amount of protein. All fats are high in calories (9 calories per gram) and should be carefully measured. It is advisable to modify fat intake by eating unsaturated fats instead of saturated fats. The sodium content of these foods varies widely (e.g., nuts can be purchased salted or unsalted), so you will need to check the food label for sodium information.

Unsaturated Fats

Avocado	⅛ medium
Margarine	1 Tsp
☒ Margarine, diet	1 Tbsp
Mayonnaise	1 Tsp
☒ Mayonnaise (reduced-calorie)	1 Tbsp

Nuts, Seeds, and Olives

Almonds, dry roasted	6
Cashews, dry roasted	1 Tbsp
Pecans	2
Peanuts (small)	20
Peanuts (large)	10
Walnuts	2 whole
Other nuts	1 Tbsp
Seeds (except pumpkin), including pine nuts and sunflower seeds (without shells)	1 Tbsp
Pumpkin seeds	2 Tsp
☒ Olives (small)	10
☒ Olives (large)	5

Salad Dressings and Oils

Oil (corn, cottonseed, safflower, soybean, sunflower, olive, peanut)	1 Tsp
Salad dressing, mayonnaise-type, regular	2 Tsp
Salad dressing, mayonnaise-type, reduced-calorie	1 Tbsp
Salad dressing, all varieties, regular	1 Tbsp
☒ Salad dressing, reduced-calorie (low-cal is free)	2 Tbsp

Saturated Fats	
Butter	1 Tsp
☒ Bacon	1 slice
Chitterlings	½ oz
Coconut, shredded	2 Tbsp
Coffee creamer, liquid	2 Tbsp
Coffee creamer, powder	4 Tsp
Cream (light, coffee)	2 Tbsp
Cream, sour	2 Tbsp
Cream (heavy, whipping)	1 Tbsp
Cream cheese	1 Tbsp
☒ Salt pork	¼ oz

Free Foods

A free food is any food or drink that contains fewer than 20 calories per serving. In addition, your family can eat as much as you want of items that have no serving size specified, but eat only 2 to 3 servings per day of those items that have a specific serving size and spread them out throughout the day.

Seasonings can be very helpful in making foods taste better, but be careful of how much sodium you use. Read labels to help you choose seasonings without excessive amounts of sodium or salt.

Drinks	
☒ Bouillon or broth without fat	
Bouillon, low-sodium	
Carbonated drinks, sugar-free	
Carbonated water	
Club soda	

Cocoa powder, unsweetened	1 Tbsp
Coffee/tea (black)	
Drink mixes, sugar-free	
Tonic water, sugar-free	

Fruit	
Cranberries, unsweetened	½ cup
Rhubarb, unsweetened	½ cup

Vegetables (raw, 1 cup)	
Cabbage	
Celery	
☒ Chinese cabbage	
Cucumber	
Green onion	
Hot peppers	
Mushrooms	
Radishes	
☒ Zucchini	
Salad greens	
Endive	
Escarole	
Lettuce	
Romaine	
Spinach	

Sweets	
Candy, hard, sugar-free	
Gelatin, sugar-free	
Gum, sugar-free	

Jam/jelly, sugar-free	(2 Tsp)
Pancake syrup, sugar-free	(1–2 Tbsp)
Sugar substitutes (saccharin, aspartame)	
Whipped topping	(2 Tbsp)

Condiments

Catsup	(1 Tbsp)
Horseradish	
Mustard	
Nonstick pan spray	
☒ Pickles, dill, unsweetened	
Salad dressing, low-calorie	(2 Tbsp)
Taco sauce	(1 Tbsp)
Vinegar	

Seasonings

Basil (fresh)	Lemon pepper
Celery seed	Lime
Cinnamon	Lime juice
Chili powder	Mint
Chives	Onion powder
Curry	Oregano
Dill	Paprika
Flavoring extracts (vanilla, almond, etc.)	Pepper
Garlic	Pimento
Garlic powder	☒ Soy sauce
Herbs	Soy sauce, low-sodium ("lite")
Hot pepper sauce	Wine, used in cooking (¼ cup)
Lemon	Worcestershire sauce
Lemon juice	

Combination Foods

Much of the food we eat is mixed together in various combinations rather than eaten alone. Such foods do not fit into only one exchange list as it can be quite hard to tell what is in a certain casserole dish or baked food item. The following is a list of average values for some typical combination foods:

Food	Amount	Exchanges
Casserole, homemade	1 cup (8 oz)	2 medium-fat meat, 2 starches, 1 fat
☒ Cheese pizza, thin crust	¼ of a 10-inch pizza	1 medium-fat meat, 2 starches, 1 fat
☺ ☒ Chili with beans (commercial)	1 cup (8 oz)	2 medium-fat meat, 2 starches, 2 fats
☺ ☒ Chow mein (no noodles or rice)	2 cups (16 oz)	2 lean meat, 1 starch, 2 vegetables
☒ Macaroni and cheese	1 cup (8 oz)	1 medium-fat meat, 2 starches, 2 fats
Soups		
☺ ☒ Bean	1 cup (8 oz)	1 lean meat, 1 starch, 1 vegetable
☒ Chunky, all varieties	10¾-oz can	1 medium-fat meat, 1 starch, 1 vegetable
☒ Cream (canned, made with water)	1 cup (8 oz)	1 starch, 1 fat
☒ Vegetable or broth	1 cup (8 oz)	1 starch
☒ Spaghetti and meatballs (canned)	1 cup (8 oz)	1 medium-fat meat, 1 fat, 2 starches
Sugar-free pudding (with skim milk)	¼ cup	1 starch
If beans are used as a meat substitute		
☺ Dried beans, peas, lentils	1 cup (cooked)	1 lean meat, 2 starches

Foods for Occasional Use

According to the exchanges, moderate amounts of some foods can be used in your meal plan, in spite of their sugar or fat content, as long as you can maintain blood glucose control. The following list includes average exchange values for some of these foods; as they are concentrated sources of carbohydrate, you will notice that the portion sizes are very small.

Food	Amount	Exchanges
Angel-food cake	½ cake	2 starches
Cake, no icing	½ cake (3-inch square)	2 starches, 2 fats
Cookies	2 small (1¾ inches across)	2 starches, 1 fat
Frozen fruit yogurt	⅓ cup	1 starch
Gingersnaps	3	1 starch
Granola	¼ cup	1 starch, 1 fat
Granola bars	1 small	1 starch, 1 fat
Ice cream, any flavor	½ cup	1 starch, 2 fats
Ice milk, any flavor	½ cup	1 starch, 1 fat
Sherbet, any flavor	¼ cup	1 starch
☒ Snack chips, all varieties	1 oz	1 starch, 2 fats
Vanilla wafers	6 small	1 starch, 2 fats

Measurement of Foods

It is important to eat the right serving sizes of food, so you will need to learn how to estimate the amounts of food. You can do this by measuring all the food your family eats for a week or so. Measure liquids and certain solid foods (e.g., tuna, cottage cheese, and canned fruits) with a measuring cup. Use measuring spoons for oil, salad dressing, and peanut butter. In addition, a scale can be very useful for measuring almost anything, especially meat, poultry, and fish. All food should be measured or weighed after cooking since many foods will weigh less after you cook them (particularly meats). Starchy foods like rice often swell in cooking, so a small amount of uncooked starch will become a much larger amount of cooked food. The following table shows some of the expected changes:

Starch Group	Uncooked	Cooked
Oatmeal	3 level Tbsp	½ cup
Cream of Wheat	2 level Tbsp	½ cup
Grits	3 level Tbsp	½ cup
Rice	2 level Tbsp	½ cup
Spaghetti	¼ cup	½ cup
Noodles	⅓ cup	½ cup
Macaroni	¼ cup	½ cup
Dried beans	3 Tbsp	⅓ cup
Dried peas	3 Tbsp	⅓ cup
Lentils	2 Tbsp	⅓ cup
Meat Group		
Hamburger	4 oz	3 oz
Chicken	1 small drumstick	1 oz
Chicken	½ of a whole chicken breast	3 oz

APPENDIX C:
PHYSICAL ACTIVITY, NUTRITION,
AND DIABETES WEB SITES OF INTEREST

American Council on Exercise (ACE)
www.acefitness.org/fitfacts/

American Diabetes Association (ADA)
Home page: www.diabetes.org
Club Ped: www.diabetes.org/ClubPed/index.jsp
(pedometer walking club)

American Dietetic Association (ADA)
www.eatright.org/public

America on the Move (national initiative to improve health
and quality of life)
www.americaonthemove.org

Anorexia Nervosa and Related Eating Disorders, Inc. (ANRED)
www.anred.com

Centers for Disease Control and Prevention (CDC)
Diabetes facts: www.cdc.gov/health/diabetes.htm
Growth charts: www.cdc.gov/nchs/about/major/nhanes/
growthcharts/clinical_charts.htm
Overweight and obesity: www.cdc.gov/nccdphp/dnpa/
obesity/index.htm

Center for Nutrition Policy and Promotion (CNPP)
Home page: www.cnpp.usda.gov
Interactive Healthy Eating Index and Physical Activity Tool:
http://209.48.219.53/

Center for Science in the Public Interest (*Nutrition Action* newsletter)
www.cspinet.org

Children with Diabetes (online community and information)
www.childrenwithdiabetes.com

Diabetes Exercise and Sports Association (DESA)
www.diabetes-exercise.org

Diabetes in Control (research updates)
www.diabetesincontrol.com

The Diabetes Mall (diabetes supplies and helpful information)
www.diabetesnet.com

Glycemic Index Information and Database (University of Sydney)
www.glycemicindex.com

Keep Kids Healthy (a pediatrician's guide to healthy kids)
Home page: www.keepkidshealthy.com

BMI calculator: www.keepkidshealthy.com/welcome/
bmicalculator.html

National Institutes of Health (NIH)
Facts about dietary supplements: www.cc.nih.gov/ccc/
supplements/

The President's Challenge (physical activity and fitness awards
program)
Home page: www.presidentschallenge.org
BMI calculator: www.presidentschallenge.org/tools_to_help/
bmi.aspx

The President's Council on Physical Fitness and Sports
Home page: www.fitness.gov
Fitness handbook: www.fitness.gov/getfit.pdf (for youth ages six to
seventeen)

Shape Up America (nonprofit group dedicated to achieving a healthy
weight for life)
www.shapeup.org

TransFreeAmerica (national campaign to eliminate partially hydrogenated oils)
www.transfreeamerica.org

Tufts University Nutrition Navigator (rating guide to nutrition
Web sites)
www:navigator.tufts.edu

U.S. Food and Drug Administration (FDA)
Dietary supplements: www.cfsan.fda.gov/~dms/supplmnt.html
Nutrient database search: www.nal.usda.gov/fnic/foodcomp/
search/

SELECTED REFERENCES

Introduction

American Diabetes Association (2000). Type 2 diabetes in children and adolescents. *Diabetes Care*, 23: 381–89.

Fagot-Campagna, A. (2000). Emergence of type 2 diabetes in children: the epidemiological evidence. *Journal of Pediatric Endocrinology and Metabolism*, 13: 1394–1402.

Narayan, K., J. Boyle, T. Thompson, S. Sorensen, and D. Williamson (2003). Lifetime risk for diabetes mellitus in the United States. *Journal of the American Medical Association*, 290: 1884–90.

Rosenbloom A., J. Joe, R. Young, and W. Winter (1999). Emerging epidemic of type 2 diabetes in youth. *Diabetes Care*, 22: 345–54.

Chapter 1

American Diabetes Association (2003). Clinical practice recommendations: Report of the expert committee on the diagnosis and classification of diabetes mellitus. *Diabetes Care,* 26 (Suppl. 1): S5–S20.

American Diabetes Association (2000). Type 2 diabetes in children and adolescents. *Diabetes Care,* 23: 381–89.

Berggren, J., M. Hulver, G. Dohm, and J. Houmard (2004). Weight loss and exercise: Implications for muscle lipid metabolism and insulin action. *Medicine & Science in Sports & Exercise,* 36: 1191–95.

Bruce, C., and J. Hawley (2004). Improvements in insulin resistance with aerobic exercise training: A lipocentric approach. *Medicine & Science in Sports & Exercise,* 36: 1196–1201.

Centers for Disease Control and Prevention (2000). National Diabetes Fact Sheet: General information and national estimates on diabetes in the United States, 2000. Retrieved from www.cdc.gov/diabetes/pubs/estimates.htm.

Centers for Disease Control and Prevention (October 24, 2002). Prevalence of overweight among children and adolescents: United States, 1999–2000. Retrieved from www.cdc.gov/nchs/products/pubs/pubd/hestats/overwght99.htm.

DiabetesInControl.com (May 19, 2004). Across the globe 1 in 10 schoolchildren are overweight. Retrieved from www.diabetesincontrol.com/issue208/item7.shtml.

Fukagawa, N., J. Anderson, G. Hageman, V. Young, and K. Minaker (1990). High-carbohydrate, high-fiber diets increase peripheral insulin sensitivity in healthy young and old adults. *American Journal of Clinical Nutrition,* 52: 524–28.

Gaesser, G. (2002). *Big, Fat Lies: The Truth About Your Weight and Your Health* (updated edition). Carlsbad, CA: Gürze Books.

Tuomilehto, J., J. Lindstrom, J. G. Eriksson, et al. (2001). Prevention of type 2 diabetes mellitus by changes in lifestyle among subjects with impaired glucose tolerance. *New England Journal of Medicine,* 344: 1343–50.

Chapter 2

American Diabetes Association (2003). Clinical practice recommendations: Evidence-based nutrition principles and recommendations for the treatment and prevention of diabetes and related complications. *Diabetes Care,* 26 (Suppl. 1): S51–S61.

Brand-Miller, J., S. Hayne, P. Petocz, and S. Colagiuri (2003). Low-glycemic index diets in the management of diabetes: A meta-analysis of randomized control trials. *Diabetes Care,* 26: 2261–67.

Foster-Powell, K., S. Holt, and J. Brand-Miller (2002). International table of glycemic index and glycemic load values: 2002. *American Journal of Clinical Nutrition,* 76: 5–56.

Goudswaard, A., R. Stalk, H. de Valk, and G. Rutten (2003). Improving glycemic control in patients with type 2 diabetes mellitus without insulin therapy. *Diabetic Medicine,* 20: 540–44.

Jenkins, D., C. Kendall, A. Marchie, et al. (2003). Type 2 diabetes and the vegetarian diet. *American Journal of Clinical Nutrition,* 78: 610S–16S.

Liu, R. (2003). Health benefits of fruit and vegetables are from additive and synergistic combinations of phytochemicals. *American Journal of Clinical Nutrition,* 78: 517S–20S.

Lovejoy, J. (2002). The influence of dietary fat on insulin resistance. *Current Diabetes Reports,* 2: 435–40.

Reynolds, L., and M. Finke (2002). The influence of sweetened drink consumption on the likelihood of meeting the recommended dietary allowance for vitamins and minerals. *Family and Consumer Sciences Research Journal,* 31(2): 195–205.

Rizkalla, S., L. Taghrid, M. Laromiguiere, et al. (2004). Improved plasma glucose control, whole-body glucose utilization, and lipid profile on a low-glycemic index diet in type 2 diabetic men. *Diabetes Care,* 27: 1866–72.

Willett, W., J. Manson, and S. Liu (2002). Glycemic index, glycemic load, and risk of type 2 diabetes. *American Journal of Clinical Nutrition,* 76 (Suppl.): 274S–80S.

Chapter 3

Field, A. E., S. B. Austin, C. B. Taylor, et al. (2003). Relation between dieting and weight change among pre-adolescents and adolescents. *Pediatrics,* 112: 900–06.

James, J., and D. Kerr (2003). Implicating sugar-sweetened soda in the aetiology of childhood obesity. *Diabetes,* 52: A70.

USDA's Center for Nutrition Policy and Promotion (2004). The food guide pyramid. Retrieved from www.pueblo.gsa.gov/cic_text /food/food-pyramid/main.html.

Yeoman, B. (June 2003). Is the food pyramid making you fat? *Fitness,* 133–36.

Chapter 4

American College of Sports Medicine (2000). Exercise and type 2 diabetes. *Medicine & Science in Sports & Exercise,* 32: 1345–60.

American Diabetes Association (2003). Clinical practice recommendations: Diabetes mellitus and exercise. *Diabetes Care,* 26 (Suppl. 1): S73–S77.

Borghouts, L, and H. Keizer (2000). Exercise and insulin sensitivity: a review. *International Journal of Sports Medicine,* 21: 1–12.

Kriska, A. (2003). Can a physically active lifestyle prevent type 2 diabetes? *Exercise and Sport Sciences Reviews,* 31: 132–37.

Larsen, J., F. Dela, S. Madsbad, J. Vibe-Petersen, and H. Galbo (1999). Interaction of sulfonylureas and exercise on glucose homeostasis in type 2 diabetic patients. *Diabetes Care,* 22: 1647–54.

McCabe, M., and L. Ricciardelli (2003). Body image and strategies to lose weight and increase muscle among boys and girls. *Health Psychology,* 22: 39–46.

Stevens, J., J. Cai, K. Evenson, and R. Thomas (2002). Fitness and fatness as predictors of morality from all causes and from cardiovascular disease in men and women in the Lipid Research Clinics Study. *American Journal of Epidemiology,* 156: 832–41.

Wing, R., and J. Hill (2001). Successful weight loss maintenance. *Annual Reviews in Nutrition,* 21: 323–41.

Chapter 5

Hale, B. (2001). Get Fit! A handbook for youth ages 6–17: How to get in shape to meet the President's challenge. President's Council on Physical Fitness and Sports. Retrieved from www.presidentschallenge.org/pdf/getfit.pdf.

Hayes, C. (2000). *The "I Hate To Exercise" Book for People with Diabetes.* Alexandria, VA: American Diabetes Association.

Hornsby, G., Jr., editor in chief (1994). *The Fitness Book for People with Diabetes: A Project of the American Diabetes Association Council on Exercise.* Alexandria, VA: American Diabetes Association.

Hu, F., T. Li, and W. Willett, et al. (2003). Television watching and other sedentary behaviors in relation to risk of obesity and type 2 diabetes mellitus in women. *Journal of the American Medical Association,* 289: 1785–91.

Hu, F., R. Sigal, and J. Rich-Edwards, et al. (1999). Walking compared with vigorous physical activity and risk of type 2 diabetes in women: A prospective study. *Journal of the American Medical Association,* 282: 1433–39.

Price, J. (2003). *The Anytime, Anywhere Exercise Book.* Avon, MA: Adams Media Corporation.

Saris, W., S. Blair, M. van Baak, et al. (2003). How much physical activity is enough to prevent unhealthy weight gain? Outcome of the IASO First Stock Conference and consensus statement. *Obesity Reviews,* 4: 101–14.

U.S. Department of Health and Human Services (2000). Physical activity and health: A report of the Surgeon General Executive Committee. Retrieved from www.fitness.gov/execsum.htm.

Chapter 6

Chausmer, A. (1998). Zinc, insulin and diabetes. *Journal of the American College of Nutrition,* 17: 109–15.

Chiu, K., A. Chu, V. Go, and M. Saad (2004). Low vitamin D worsens beta cell function. *American Journal of Clinical Nutrition,* 79: 820–25.

Cusi, K., S. Cukier, R. DeFronzo, et al. (2001). Vanadyl sulfate improves hepatic and muscle insulin sensitivity in type 2 diabetes. *Journal of Clinical Endocrinology and Metabolism,* 86: 1410–17.

Ruhe, R., and R. McDonald (2001). Use of antioxidant nutrients in the prevention and treatment of type 2 diabetes. *Journal of the American College of Nutrition,* 20: 363S–68S.

Ryan, E., S. Imes, and C. Wallace (2001). Short-term intensity insulin therapy in newly diagnosed type 2 diabetes. *Diabetes Care,* 27: 1028–32.

Yeh, G., D. Eisenberg, T. Kaptchuk, and R. Phillips (2003). Systematic review of herbs and dietary supplements for glycemic control in diabetes. *Diabetes Care,* 26: 1277–94.

SUGGESTED READINGS

Barnes, D., and American College of Sports Medicine (2004). *Action Plan for Diabetes: Your Guide to Controlling Blood Sugar.* Champaign, IL: Human Kinetics.

Brand-Miller, J., et al. (2003). *The New Glucose Revolution.* New York: Marlowe & Company.

Bricklin, M., and L. Konner (1995). *Prevention's Your Perfect Weight: The Diet-Free Weight-Loss Method Developed by the World's Leading Health Magazine.* Emmaus, PA: Rodale Press, Inc.

Chous, A. (2003). *Diabetic Eye Disease: Lessons from a Diabetic Eye Doctor. How to Avoid Blindness and Get Great Eye Care.* Auburn, WA: Fairwood Press, Inc.

Colberg, S. (2001). *The Diabetic Athlete: Prescriptions for Exercise and Sports.* Champaign, IL: Human Kinetics.

Cooper, K. (1999). *Fit Kids! The Complete Shape-up Program from Birth Through High School.* Nashville, TN: Broadman & Holman Publishers.

Friesz, M. (2002). *Food, Fun n' Fitness: Designing Healthy Lifestyles for Our Children.* Boca Raton, FL: Designs for Healthy Lifestyles Publishing.

Gaesser, G. (2002). *Big, Fat Lies: The Truth About Your Weight and Your Health* (updated edition). Carlsbad, CA: Gürze Books.

Goleman, D. (1995). *Emotional Intelligence: Why It Can Matter More than IQ.* New York: Bantam Books.

Hayes, C. (2000). *The "I Hate to Exercise" Book for People with Diabetes.* Alexandria, VA: American Diabetes Association.

Hornsby, G., Jr., editor in chief (1994). *The Fitness Book for People with Diabetes: A Project of the American Diabetes Association Council on Exercise.* Alexandria, VA: American Diabetes Association.

Joseph, J., D. Nadeau, and A. Underwood (2003). *The Color Code: A Revolutionary Eating Plan for Optimal Health.* New York: Hyperion.

Price, J. (2003). *The Anytime, Anywhere Exercise Book.* Avon, MA: Adams Media Corporation.

Rosenbloom, A., J. Silverstein, and E. Baldwin (2003). *Managing Type 2 Diabetes in Children and Adolescents.* Boston: McGraw-Hill/Contemporary Books.

Ruderman, N., editor in chief (2002). *Handbook of Exercise in Diabetes.* Alexandria, VA: American Diabetes Association.

Shield, J., and M. Mullen (2002). *American Dietetic Association Guide to Healthy Eating for Kids: How Your Children Can Eat Smart from Five to Twelve.* Hoboken, NJ: Wiley.

Warshaw, H. (2002). *Guide to Healthy Restaurant Eating,* 2nd edition. Boston: McGraw-Hill/Contemporary Books.

Williams, M. (2004). *Nutrition for Health, Fitness, and Sport,* 7th edition. Boston: McGraw-Hill.

INDEX

ABOUT THE AUTHORS

Sheri Colberg, Ph.D., received her doctorate from the University of California at Berkeley. She is an exercise physiologist and associate professor of exercise science at Old Dominion University in Norfolk, Virginia. A diabetic herself, she specializes in diabetes and exercise, conducting extensive clinical research in diabetes and exercise with funding from the American Diabetes Association and others. She has also authored more than fifty articles on exercise and diabetes, as well as *The Diabetic Athlete* (Human Kinetics, 2001), translated into Japanese, Portuguese, and Spanish.

A frequent lecturer on diabetes and physical activity, Dr. Colberg is also a reviewer for many scientific journals, a member of diabetes advisory boards, an exercise adviser for dLife, a fellow of the American

College of Sports Medicine, a professional member of the American Diabetes Association, and a member of Marquis *Who's Who in America.*

Dr. Colberg currently resides in Virginia Beach, Virginia, with her husband and their three boys, who have given her more than a decade's worth of practical parenting experience. An avid recreational exerciser, she enjoys swimming, biking, walking, fitness machines, tennis, racquetball, weight training, hiking, and yard work, as well as playing with her three active sons.

Visit Dr. Colberg's Web site at www.SheriColberg.com, or e-mail her at Sheri@SheriColberg.com.

Mary Friesz, Ph.D., R.D., is a registered and licensed dietitian with a degree in nutrition and exercise physiology from Columbia University. A certified diabetes educator (CDE), she also has a Ph.D. in social psychology and twenty years' experience in health and fitness, which she puts to use in her nutrition and wellness consulting practice, Designs for Healthy Lifestyles. Recently focusing on youth with "diabesity" and eating disorders, she is sensitive to the special needs of children. In spite of having suffered from obesity as a child and eating disorders as an adolescent, she has maintained a healthy lifestyle for more than two decades. Ms. Friesz is also a professional speaker, a developer of course curricula and continuing education programs, and an adjunct professor at the University of Phoenix. She currently resides in south Florida with her son.